INCLUDES 14 MEA[...]
ALL UNDER 20g NE[...]

200 UNDER 20g NET CARBS

200 KETO DIET-FRIENDLY RECIPES to Keep You UNDER 20g NET CARBS Every Day!

Lindsay Boyers, CHNC

Adams Media
New York · London · Toronto · Sydney · New Delhi

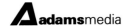

Adams Media
An Imprint of Simon & Schuster, Inc.
57 Littlefield Street
Avon, Massachusetts 02322

First Adams Media trade paperback edition August 2020

ADAMS MEDIA and colophon are trademarks of Simon & Schuster.

For information about special discounts for bulk purchases, please contact Simon & Schuster Special Sales at 1-866-506-1949 or business@simonandschuster.com.

The Simon & Schuster Speakers Bureau can bring authors to your live event. For more information or to book an event contact the Simon & Schuster Speakers Bureau at 1-866-248-3049 or visit our website at www.simonspeakers.com.

Interior design by Sylvia McArdle
Photographs by James Stefiuk; © 123RF/Oksana Mironova, Seksak Kerdkanno;
Getty Images/Floortje

Manufactured in the United States of America

10 9 8 7 6 5 4 3 2 1

Library of Congress Cataloging-in-Publication Data
Names: Boyers, Lindsay, author.
Title: 200 under 20g net carbs / Lindsay Boyers, CHNC.
Description: First Adams Media trade paperback edition. | Avon, Massachusetts: Adams Media, 2020. | Includes index.
Identifiers: LCCN 2020008677 | ISBN 9781507213919 (pb) | ISBN 9781507213926 (ebook)
Subjects: LCSH: Low-carbohydrate diet--Recipes. | Ketogenic diet--Recipes. | LCGFT: Cookbooks.
Classification: LCC RM237.73 .B6917 2020 | DDC 641.5/6383--dc23
LC record available at https://lccn.loc.gov/2020008677

ISBN 978-1-5072-1391-9
ISBN 978-1-5072-1392-6 (ebook)

Contains material adapted from the following titles published by Adams Media, an Imprint of Simon & Schuster, Inc.: *The Everything® Ketogenic Diet Cookbook* by Lindsay Boyers, CHNC, copyright © 2017, ISBN 978-1-5072-0626-3; *The Everything® Keto Diet Meal Prep Cookbook* by Lindsay Boyers, CHNC, copyright © 2019, ISBN 978-1-5072-1045-1; *The Everything® Keto Cycling Cookbook* by Lindsay Boyers, CHNC, copyright © 2019, ISBN 978-1-5072-1059-8; and *The Everything® Low-Carb Meal Prep Cookbook* by Lindsay Boyers, CHNC, copyright © 2018, ISBN 978-1-5072-0731-4.

CONTENTS

CHAPTER 9

SIDE DISHES 175

CHAPTER 10

FAT BOMBS 194

CHAPTER 11

SWEETS AND TREATS 218

INTRODUCTION

One of the first questions that pops up when discussing the keto diet is: "How many carbs can you eat?" While there are many factors that can influence your individual goals, there is a standard "sweet spot" that tends to work really well across the board: 20 grams of net carbs per day. But it can be difficult to find a variety of recipes with low net carb counts—that's where *200 under 20g Net Carbs* comes in! This book gives you a whopping two hundred recipes—including breakfast, snacks, soups and salads, dinner entrées, meatless meals, side dishes, and plenty of desserts—all of which are designed to keep you at 20 grams or less of net carbs per day.

Counting net carbs isn't as difficult as it might sound. This book explains the basics of the keto lifestyle so you can get started as quickly as possible, then gives you two hundred recipes that include easy-to-follow steps and a full nutritional panel. You'll also find two weeks' worth of strategically designed meal plans that make transitioning to a keto diet simple and straightforward. If you're someone who likes to have a strict plan or you're new to a keto diet and need clear guidance, you can follow the meal plans exactly as they're written. If you prefer a little more freedom, or you're already a keto pro and you're just looking for some new ideas to add to your meal plans, you can mix and match the recipes in the meal plans based on your own preferences and dietary needs.

Best of all, you don't have to sacrifice any flavor or taste to stay under 20 grams a day. Whether you're savoring Bacon Cheddar Chive Biscuits for breakfast, snacking on Spicy Chili Kale Chips, whipping up Garlic Feta–Baked Chicken Thighs for dinner, or enjoying Double Chocolate Mousse Bars for a treat, you'll stay on track to meet your goals with these mouthwatering recipes!

CHAPTER 1

COUNTING CARBS

The keto diet is built off of one major principle: counting carbs. Yes, it's also about optimizing your nutrition by eating plenty of healthy fats, nutrient-dense vegetables, and high-quality proteins. But being aware of how many carbs you're eating on a daily basis is the key to seeing the enormous benefits. The good news is that counting carbs is actually really easy and straightforward once you get the hang of it.

THE BASICS OF A KETO DIET

A ketogenic diet focuses on reducing the number of carbohydrates (especially sugar and grains) you eat, while consuming protein and a high amount of fat. The ultimate goal of the keto diet is to restrict carbohydrates enough that you kick your body into ketosis—a metabolic state in which your body burns fat for energy instead of carbohydrates.

Before jumping into how to count carbs, it's advantageous if you know why you're cutting carbs in the first place. (Sometimes it's easier to stick to something for the long term if you know why you're doing it.) When it comes to the keto diet, it's important to understand exactly how carbs affect your body physiologically, the physical benefits of scaling back on the amount of carbs you consume, and why you should be discerning about the type you eat.

The Benefits of Cutting Carbs

Lots of people start a keto diet with weight loss as the main motivating factor. But while shedding pounds is certainly a worthy goal—and something that will improve your health in general—the benefits of keto go way beyond weight loss. Unlike diets that focus solely on calorie restriction, a well-designed, nutritionally balanced keto diet can also:

- Boost energy levels
- Change body composition (less fat and more muscle)
- Decrease inflammation
- Improve brain function (better concentration, less brain fog, better memory, etc.)
- Lower blood sugar levels and improve insulin sensitivity
- Reduce risk factors for heart disease (cholesterol levels, blood pressure, and blood sugar)
- Alleviate anxiety and depression

- Slow tumor growth for some cancers
- Minimize symptoms of Alzheimer's and slow disease progression
- Reduce frequency and severity of seizures in those with epilepsy

Cutting out carbohydrates—especially simple ones, like sugar and refined flour—also helps balance your hormones, which really control what's going on in the rest of your body.

WHAT HAPPENS WHEN YOU OVEREAT CARBS

When you eat carbohydrates, your body's goal is to break them down into their simplest form, which is glucose. When glucose moves into the bloodstream, it triggers the pancreas to release the hormone insulin. In this instance, insulin's job is to attach to glucose and carry it into your cells, where it's used as an energy source. After your body uses up all of the energy it needs, it will turn some of the remaining glucose into glycogen, which is a storage form of glucose. That glycogen is then stored in your muscles or your liver.

But your body's ability to store glycogen isn't unlimited. There's a point when glycogen stores fill up, and your muscles and liver just can't hold any more. At this point, the glycogen that's left over gets turned into fatty acids. This isn't a problem in and of itself, but it becomes a problem if you're not later using any of those fatty acids for energy, because your body will continue to store them.

Some of these fatty acids are stored in your fat tissues, but others are stored in your liver, and some are converted into triglycerides and circulated through your body in your blood. The more carbohydrates you overeat, the higher your fatty acid and triglyceride numbers get. Over time, high triglycerides can cause heart disease, heart attacks, and problems with your liver and pancreas. Excess simple carbohydrate consumption is actually one of the main underlying causes of nonalcoholic fatty liver disease.

WHERE FAT IS STORED

Your body has a limited ability to store carbohydrates. It uses the glucose it needs and then stores about twenty-four hours' worth of glycogen, the storage form of glucose, in the liver for use in between meals. On the other hand, your body's ability to store fat is endless. If your fat cells run out of room, your body will just make them bigger so it can store more fat. Over time, this process can contribute to weight gain.

The keto diet discourages that overflow of carbohydrates. Your body prioritizes using carbohydrates for energy, but in their absence, it will turn to fat—its second-favorite source—for the fuel it needs. To turn fat into usable energy, the liver breaks down fatty acids into energy-rich substances called *ketones*. When your body is creating ketones, you're in a state of ketosis—or in other words, your body is burning fat for energy instead of carbohydrates. That's how the keto diet helps you use up excess fatty acid reserves.

WHAT IS INSULIN RESISTANCE?

The hormone insulin plays a significant role in how your body processes carbs. The type and amount of carbohydrates you eat also has a major impact on that process. Simple carbohydrates like white sugar and white flour are broken down quickly and, as a result, glucose rushes into the bloodstream. This rush of glucose triggers a rapid release of insulin. Once the insulin attaches to the glucose and carries it to your cells, your blood sugar levels drop quickly. These highs and lows don't have too much of a negative impact if they happen only occasionally, but if they happen all the time, it can have a long-term negative effect on your overall health and your mood.

Over time, this blood sugar roller coaster can also lead to insulin resistance, which increases the risk of long-term health problems, like prediabetes, type 2 diabetes, heart attacks, stroke, and even cancer.

cose. After digestion, fats become free fatty acids, and proteins become amino acids. While protein can raise your blood sugar slightly (depending on what the rest of your diet looks like), fat doesn't affect it at all. If your blood sugar isn't rising, your body isn't prompted to release insulin. And when you keep your blood sugar levels steady for an extended length of time, this allows all of the other hormones in your body to balance themselves out naturally.

ARE YOU INSULIN RESISTANT?

Insulin resistance is a problem that plagues one in three Americans (one in two age sixty or older). It's often dubbed a silent problem because many people don't even know they have it until it progresses to type 2 diabetes. Some of the tell-tale signs of insulin resistance are increased thirst or hunger, frequent urination, tingling sensations in your hands and feet, and feeling more tired than usual. People with insulin resistance also tend to carry a lot of their extra weight in their belly. If you suspect that you're insulin resistant, ask your doctor to test your LP-IR score. Many doctors use blood sugar to determine diabetes risk, but by the time insulin resistance negatively affects blood sugar, it's a problem that's been going on for years.

WILL PROTEIN KICK YOU OUT OF KETOSIS?

A lot of people think eating too much protein will kick you out of ketosis, but how protein affects your blood sugar and insulin depends on what the rest of your diet looks like. In the absence of carbohydrates, protein only raises the level of a hormone called glucagon, which helps you burn fat. When you combine protein with carbohydrates, insulin and glucagon go up. When both hormone levels increase, insulin overpowers glucagon and promotes fat storage instead.

There are indirect hormonal benefits of restricting carbohydrates too. Naturally, when you remove something from your diet, you have to replace it with something else. On the keto diet, healthy fat sources replace the unhealthy carbohydrate sources that you remove. These "good" fats—which come from avocados, olive oil, coconut oil, and yes, even butter—act as the building blocks for important sex hormones, like estrogen, progesterone, and testosterone.

When you focus on eating mostly fat and some high-quality proteins, you take away the trigger that starts this undesirable cascade of events: glucose. Carbohydrates are the only macronutrient that gets broken down into glu-

THE MACRONUTRIENT BREAKDOWN

What is the sweet spot for how much carbs, fat, and protein to eat to prevent insulin spikes? The exact macronutrient breakdown can vary from person to person, but in general, a keto diet typically looks something like this:

- 60–75 percent of calories from fat
- 15–30 percent of calories from protein
- 5–10 percent of calories from carbohydrates

There's no one-size-fits-all approach to a well-designed keto plan, but a few generalities seem to work well across the board. While some people can get away with eating up to 50 grams of net carbs per day, when making generalized recommendations, 20 grams of net carbs per day is the "sweet spot" that can get everybody (even those with insulin resistance) into ketosis.

WHAT ARE NET CARBS?

The term *net carbs* refers to the carbs that are actually absorbed by your body. When counting carbs for a keto diet, the focus is only on net carbs, not total carbs, because only net carbs have significant effects on your blood sugar and insulin levels. Since fiber and sugar alcohols don't get broken down into glucose, they don't cause blood sugar spikes and don't trigger your body to release insulin. Because of this, they're essentially "free" carbohydrates.

To calculate net carbohydrates, take the number of total carbohydrates and subtract grams of fiber and grams of sugar alcohols. The number you're left with represents the net carbs. For example, If a recipe contains 9 grams of total carbs, but 4 grams of those carbs come from fiber, the recipe has 5 grams of net carbs. If a recipe has 17 grams of total carbs, but 13 of those grams are in the form of sugar alcohols, the net carb count is 4 grams.

Fiber

Fiber is a type of carbohydrate that's resistant to human digestion. Its sugar molecules are linked in a unique way that your digestive enzymes can't break apart. Because of this, fiber passes through the digestive tract in one piece until it reaches the colon. Once the fiber gets to your colon, the good bacteria that live there start to break it down, creating short-chain fatty acids (SCFAs) in the process. These SCFAs don't affect your blood sugar or insulin levels, but they do keep your gut healthy, help you manage your weight, and may prevent type 2 diabetes. That's why fiber is an excellent carbohydrate choice for a keto diet.

YOUR SECOND BRAIN

Fiber-rich foods promote the growth of good bacteria in your gut. A balance of gut bacteria improves your health and significantly boosts your mood. In fact, gut health is such an intricate part of your mental health that researchers often call your gut your "second brain." This "second brain," which is officially called the enteric nervous system, is a collection of more than one hundred million neurons (more than both the brain and the spinal cord) that has its own reflexes and senses. In fact, researchers estimate that 90 percent of the information in the main nerve in your gut (called the vagus nerve) is carried from the gut to the brain. That means your gut likely sends messages to your brain, and not the other way around.

Sugar Alcohols

Sugar alcohols are another type of carbohydrate that are partially absorbed in the small intestine. These carbohydrates have varying effects on your blood sugar and insulin levels because some are almost immediately removed through your urine while others enter your bloodstream. There are several different types of sugar alcohols:

- Erythritol
- Isomalt
- Sorbitol
- Maltitol
- Xylitol

Although they're all subtracted from total carbohydrate counts when calculating your net carbs, erythritol is the best choice because 90 percent of it is excreted in your urine and only about 10 percent enters your colon. As a result, it doesn't affect your blood sugar at all. On the other hand, some studies show that maltitol may actually increase your blood glucose levels.

Another thing to consider is that many sugar alcohols can cause uncomfortable digestive symptoms, like gas, bloating, and diarrhea. That's because when they reach your large intestine, the bacteria that live there start breaking them down, creating gas in the process. While most sugar alcohols have this effect to some degree (the severity depends on your personal tolerance), erythritol is highly unlikely to cause any discomfort at all because it's resistant to bacterial breakdown.

Most packaged foods that are marketed as low-carb or keto use maltitol as a sweetener, but it's best to avoid it as much as possible. Use erythritol (or other sweeteners without sugar alcohols, like stevia and monk fruit) whenever possible.

CALCULATING NET CARBS

Packaged foods make counting carbs easy. They typically list total carbohydrates, fiber, and sugar alcohols. If the label lists 15 grams of carbohydrates, but the food also has 5 grams of fiber and 8 grams of sugar alcohols, the food contains 2 grams of net carbohydrates. If the packaged food item is marketed toward keto or low-carb dieters, it may even list the net carbohydrate count for you.

Most predesigned keto recipes, like the two hundred in this book, also make things easy by listing the nutrition facts per serving. To ensure that you're staying under your goal of 20 grams of net carbs per day, just follow the meal plans or mix and match recipes according to their nutrition facts. (Of course, if you change any of the ingredients in these recipes, the net carbohydrate count may be affected, so keep that in mind when making substitutions.)

Things get trickier when you have to calculate net carbs for individual food items or recipes you've created yourself. Luckily, you can find online calculators and apps you can use to plug in recipe ingredients or individual food items like string cheese or an avocado. Some of these apps, like Carb Manager, automatically give results for net carbs. Others, like MyFitnessPal, might show only a breakdown of total carbohydrates and fiber, so you'll have to do your own math to figure out net carb numbers.

DETERMINING HOW MANY NET CARBS ARE RIGHT FOR YOU

If you're brand-new to the keto diet, it's helpful to give yourself a small transition period as you reduce your carb counts, especially if you're used to eating a lot of carbohydrates. Instead of counting carbohydrates right away, start by gradually eliminating nonnutritive carbohydrate sources, like pizza, pasta, soda, desserts, and sugary snacks over a period of about two weeks. As you're slowly phasing carbohydrates out, start introducing more healthy fats, like avocado, coconut products, and full-fat dairy items into your diet.

Once your body adjusts and you've gotten used to eating fewer carbs, then you can start paying closer attention to the actual numbers and aiming for no more than 20 grams of net carbs per day. Although 20 grams of net carbs seems to be the sweet spot for many people following a keto diet, that doesn't mean that's where you have to stay forever. As your body adjusts and your hormones become balanced, it's likely that your sensitivity to insulin will increase. In other words, a keto diet has the potential to reverse insulin resistance. When this happens, you'll have more leeway in how many carbs you can eat, and you may be able to bump your numbers up to no more than 50 grams per day. But to start, and until you reach your goals, it's beneficial to stay under 20 grams of net carbs.

QUALITY COUNTS!

While the keto diet puts a lot of emphasis on the quantity of macronutrients, quality matters too, especially when it comes to carbohydrates. While you may be able to sneak in a serving of ice cream for under 20 grams of net carbs, it's not the best decision for your body. All carbohydrates (with the exception of fiber and some sugar alcohols) turn into glucose eventually, but the rate at which they move through your digestive system plays a big role in how they affect your body and your health.

There are two major groups of carbohydrates: complex and simple.

- **Complex carbohydrates** typically have a lot of fiber and, because of this, they take longer to digest than simple carbohydrates.

Your digestive system has to break down complex carbohydrates into simpler sugars before they're small enough to move into your bloodstream. Because of this, as you digest complex carbohydrates, your blood sugar levels stay fairly low and consistent.

- **Simple carbohydrates** are generally devoid of fiber and often contain simple sugars. Because your body doesn't have to break down simple sugars to absorb them, the sugars move from your digestive tract into your bloodstream pretty quickly. This causes spikes (and resulting crashes) in both blood sugar and insulin levels. This blood sugar roller coaster can prompt your body to store extra fat, especially in your stomach area.

But these are not the only reasons complex carbohydrates are a better option. Complex carbohydrates also tend to be higher than simple carbohydrates in lots of different nutrients, like fiber, vitamins, minerals, phytonutrients, and antioxidants. When you focus on getting the majority of your 20 grams of net carbohydrates only from complex carbohydrate sources, like vegetables, you'll naturally optimize the amount and type of nutrients you're taking in.

Aside from paying attention to the types of carbohydrates you're eating, the overall quality of your food is important. There's a popular saying that "you are what you eat," but Michael Pollan, the author of *In Defense of Food*, said it better when he pointed out that "you are what what you eat eats, too." Do your best to get the highest quality food you can find and/or afford. Ideally, you want to choose meats that are organic, grass fed, and/or pasture raised. Choose grass-fed butter and organic creams, cheeses, vegetables, and fruits. Eating conventional foods won't prevent you from entering a ketogenic state, but high-quality foods are better for your body in general.

FOLLOWING THE MEAL PLANS

The meal plans at the back of this book are designed to make your life easier. Instead of memorizing lists of foods to eat and foods to avoid, trying to calculate the nutrition facts for your own recipes, or scrambling to do math in your head before you eat a meal or snack, you can use the meal plans, which are already perfectly designed to provide 20 grams or less of net carbohydrates each day. They take all of the guesswork out of the equation. All you have to do is cook them as written—and enjoy. Each day includes breakfast, lunch, dinner, a snack, and even dessert! If you want to stay at or under 20 grams of carbohydrates daily, follow the meal plans exactly as written and easily hit your goals.

If you're looking to adjust the meal plans, feel free. Since most of the recipes in this book can be easily swapped or mixed and matched, you can create your own plans based on your personal preferences. For example, if Grilled Lamb Burgers are on the menu for dinner, but lamb isn't your thing, swap them out for Cheeseburger Meatloaf instead.

Incorporating Meal Prep

Once you've decided which meal plan to follow (or you've used the included meal plans as a guide to create a plan of your own), consider meal prepping to make your days go smoothly. Prepping your meals ahead of time is not only a time saver; it is a scientifically proven way to keep you on track. Meal prepping:

- Saves time because you can make several meals at once.
- Saves money because you buy only what you need to make the recipes you're eating, and you tend to eat all of your leftovers.
- Reduces stress levels—no more worrying about what to make for dinner that night or what to eat for lunch the next day!

- Prevents overeating because you can divide recipes into individual portions before you eat them.
- Makes veering off track less likely because you have a plan in mind ahead of time.
- Gives you control over the ingredients in your food.
- Helps you manage your hunger because you have your meals and snacks ready to go so you never have to skip meals.

The first step in meal prepping is to sit down and make a grocery list. To make things simple, divide your grocery list into categories, like produce, deli items, and canned goods. This will make it easier to find things in the store. Once you've made your list, figure out when you're going to shop and when you're going to cook. If you have time, it's helpful to set aside a whole day for shopping and cooking. That way, when you get home from the grocery store, you can jump right into prepping your meals instead of having to put all your groceries away and then take them out later when you're ready to use them.

Meal prepping is also a great time to double recipes that freeze well. If you prepare an extra meal or two every time you meal prep, you'll end up with a freezer full of homemade, keto-friendly meals that you can use on days when you're too busy to cook.

GETTING STARTED

Now that you have a solid understanding of the keto diet and how to implement it, it's time to dive into the two hundred delicious recipes and meal plans in this book. Flip around and see what entices you, or try them all. Either way, get ready to enjoy mouthwatering keto dishes!

CHAPTER 2

BREAKFAST

EGGS FLORENTINE

Serves 4

This quick breakfast dish will start your day off on the right foot. If you don't have any mascarpone cheese, you can replace it with cream cheese. The two cheeses are similar and work almost the same in recipes, but because mascarpone has a higher fat content, it is richer and creamier. (Be sure to adjust nutritional stats if you swap ingredients.)

INGREDIENTS

2 tablespoons salted grass-fed butter

1 teaspoon minced garlic

2 cups chopped fresh spinach

8 large eggs, lightly beaten

½ teaspoon sea salt

¼ teaspoon ground black pepper

¼ cup mascarpone cheese

1. Heat butter in a large skillet over medium heat. Add garlic and cook for 1 minute.

2. Stir in spinach and cook until spinach is wilted, about 3 minutes.

3. Pour eggs on top of spinach and stir quickly to incorporate ingredients. Sprinkle with salt and pepper.

4. Reduce heat to low and cover. Cook for 2 minutes or until eggs start to firm up.

5. Dollop cheese over eggs and fold into thirds. Cover and cook until eggs are completely set.

6. Remove from heat, cut into four equal portions, and serve immediately.

90-SECOND BREAD

Serves 1

Bread cravings can be one of the most challenging parts of sticking to a keto diet, but this 90-Second Bread will stop them in their tracks. You can spread butter, almond butter, or cream cheese on top after toasting—or you can use it as sandwich bread.

NET CARBS
4g

Calories: 360
Fat: 32g
Sodium: 635mg
Carbohydrates: 8g
Fiber: 4g
Sugar: 2g
Sugar alcohols: 0g
Protein: 13g

INGREDIENTS

1 tablespoon salted grass-fed butter, melted

⅓ cup almond flour

1 large egg, lightly beaten

½ teaspoon baking powder

⅛ teaspoon sea salt

⅛ teaspoon garlic powder

⅛ teaspoon onion powder

1. Combine all ingredients in an ungreased 4" round microwave-safe glass dish. Whisk until fully incorporated.

2. Microwave for 90 seconds or until mixture is set. Remove from container immediately and allow to cool for 2 minutes.

3. Slice in half and toast before serving.

EGGS IN A MUG

Serves 1

If you're short on time but need a quick way to satisfy your hunger while staying on track, these Eggs in a Mug are the perfect choice. They're ready in less than 3 minutes, and since they're served in a mug and not on a plate, you can take them with you on the go.

NET CARBS
2g

Calories: 289
Fat: 24g
Sodium: 488mg
Carbohydrates: 3g
Fiber: 1g
Sugar: 1g
Sugar alcohols: 0g
Protein: 15g

INGREDIENTS

2 large eggs

1 tablespoon grass-fed heavy cream

⅛ teaspoon sea salt

⅛ teaspoon ground black pepper

1 tablespoon shredded Cheddar cheese

1 tablespoon diced avocado

1. Add eggs, cream, salt, and pepper to an ungreased 12-ounce microwave-safe mug and whisk to combine.

2. Microwave for 30 seconds, stir, and microwave for another 30 seconds. Remove from microwave and sprinkle cheese and avocado on top.

3. Serve immediately.

BACON CHEDDAR CHIVE BISCUITS

NET CARBS
3g

Calories: 416
Fat: 38g
Sodium: 656mg
Carbohydrates: 6g
Fiber: 3g
Sugar: 2g
Sugar alcohols: 0g
Protein: 14g

Serves 8

These Bacon Cheddar Chive Biscuits will have the same macros if you use regular butter—but grass-fed butter is a better choice because it is higher in conjugated linoleic acid (CLA), which has many health benefits. Studies on animals have connected CLA to a reduced risk of heart disease, a healthier immune system, diabetes prevention, and healthier bones. CLA has also been found to help reduce body fat and increase muscle mass (a combination that leads to enhanced weight loss).

INGREDIENTS

2 cups almond flour

1 teaspoon sea salt

2 teaspoons dried chives

1 cup shredded Cheddar cheese

½ cup shredded whole milk mozzarella cheese

2 large eggs

½ cup grass-fed heavy cream

2 tablespoons salted grass-fed butter, chilled and cubed

6 slices Applegate Naturals No Sugar Bacon, cooked and chopped

1. Preheat oven to 375°F. Line a baking sheet with parchment paper and set aside.

2. Combine flour, salt, and chives in a large bowl and mix until incorporated. Stir in cheeses.

3. Add eggs and cream and stir until combined. Cut in butter, using your hands or a pastry blender. Stir in bacon pieces.

4. Divide dough into eight equal-sized portions and shape into biscuits. Arrange evenly on prepared baking sheet, about 2 inches apart.

5. Bake for 20 minutes or until biscuits are slightly browned on the outside. Remove from oven and transfer to a cooling rack.

6. Allow to cool for 10 minutes before serving.

WHERE YOU CAN FIND CLA

Full-fat dairy products are the richest dietary sources of CLA. Grass-fed cows produce milk and cream that contains double the amount of CLA that's in conventional milk and cream, and five times more CLA than butter that comes from grain-fed cows.

BACON AND EGG CHEESE SANDWICH

Serves 2

This Bacon and Egg Cheese Sandwich uses a combination of mozzarella and Cheddar cheeses as the "bread." You may have to eat it with a fork instead of your hands, but you won't have to sacrifice any flavor.

Calories: 572
Fat: 45g
Sodium: 1,181mg
Carbohydrates: 3g
Fiber: 0g
Sugar: 1g
Sugar alcohols: 0g
Protein: 38g

INGREDIENTS

1 cup shredded whole milk mozzarella cheese

½ cup shredded Cheddar cheese

4 large eggs

1 tablespoon grass-fed heavy cream

⅛ teaspoon sea salt

⅛ teaspoon ground black pepper

1 tablespoon salted grass-fed butter

4 slices Applegate Naturals No Sugar Bacon, cooked

1. Preheat oven to 400°F. Line a baking sheet with parchment paper and set aside.

2. Combine cheeses in a medium bowl and mix well. Spread cheeses out in a thin square layer on prepared baking sheet. Bake for 5 minutes.

3. While cheese is baking, combine eggs, cream, salt, and pepper in a medium bowl, and whisk well. Heat butter in a large skillet over medium heat and cook egg mixture, stirring to scramble, until eggs are set and fully cooked.

4. Remove cheese from oven and drain any excess oil. Line half of the cheese shell with cooked bacon and cover with scrambled eggs.

5. Fold cheese shell in half over eggs and bacon. Return to oven and bake for another 3 minutes.

6. Remove from oven and allow to cool for 5 minutes, then cut in half and serve.

BASIC CHAFFLES

Serves 2 (Makes 4 [4"] chaffles)

net 14.29g (handwritten)

The chaffle gets its name from the fact that it's made like a waffle, but its foundational ingredient is cheese. These Basic Chaffles have a slightly eggy taste, making them perfect for breakfast, but if you want to cover that up and use your chaffles as bread for a sandwich, you can add spices like garlic powder or onion powder to make them more savory.

Calories: 309
Fat: 23g
Sodium: 513mg
Carbohydrates: 4g
Fiber: 1g
Sugar: 1g
Sugar alcohols: 0g
Protein: 21g

INGREDIENTS

Half (handwritten)

2 large eggs   *1 egg* (handwritten)

1 cup shredded whole milk mozzarella cheese   *½ C* (handwritten)

¼ cup almond flour   *⅛ cup* (handwritten)

½ teaspoon baking powder   *¼ tsp* (handwritten)

1. Preheat a mini waffle maker.

2. Add eggs to a medium bowl and whisk lightly. Stir in cheese, flour, and baking powder.

3. Pour one-fourth of the batter into heated waffle maker. Cook for 3 minutes or until steam no longer comes out of waffle maker. Repeat with remaining batter.

4. Serve immediately.

CHEDDAR CHIVE CHAFFLES

Serves 2 (Makes 4 [4"] chaffles)

The addition of Cheddar and chives adds a savory flavor that makes these chaffles a unique breakfast option. Try spreading with some cream cheese before eating.

Calories: 339
Fat: 26g
Sodium: 522mg
Carbohydrates: 5g
Fiber: 2g
Sugar: 1g
Sugar alcohols: 0g
Protein: 21g

INGREDIENTS

2 large eggs

½ cup shredded whole milk mozzarella cheese

½ cup shredded Cheddar cheese

¼ cup almond flour

½ teaspoon baking powder

1 tablespoon dried chives

1. Preheat a mini waffle maker.

2. Add eggs to a medium bowl and whisk lightly. Stir in cheeses, flour, baking powder, and chives.

3. Pour one-fourth of the batter into heated waffle maker. Cook for 3 minutes or until steam no longer comes out of waffle maker. Repeat with remaining batter.

4. Serve immediately.

BUFFALO CHICKEN EGG CUPS

Serves 12

Buffalo chicken and egg may not be a pair that you're used to seeing, but they should be! The two come together really nicely to form a high-protein keto breakfast on the go.

INGREDIENTS

12 large eggs

1 teaspoon sea salt

¼ teaspoon ground black pepper

2 tablespoons dried chives

1 (9.75-ounce) can white chunk chicken breast, drained

½ cup Frank's RedHot Original Cayenne Pepper Sauce

¼ cup shredded Cheddar cheese

1. Preheat oven to 350°F. Spray each cup of a twelve-cup mini muffin tin with coconut oil cooking spray.

2. Whisk eggs, salt, pepper, and chives together in a large mixing bowl. Combine chicken and hot sauce in a medium bowl and toss to coat.

3. Pour equal amounts of egg mixture into each cup of the muffin tin. Spoon chicken mixture evenly in each cup. Sprinkle cheese on top.

4. Bake for 15 minutes or until eggs are set.

5. Remove from oven and allow to cool for 5 minutes, then serve warm.

SAUSAGE CREAM CHEESE PINWHEELS

Serves 12

When choosing a breakfast sausage for these pinwheels, check the ingredient list carefully and make sure there's no added sugar. Lots of store-bought breakfast sausages are maple flavored and not keto-friendly. If you're having trouble finding something at the store, you can make your own with ground pork.

Calories: 265
Fat: 22g
Sodium: 405mg
Carbohydrates: 5g
Fiber: 2g
Sugar: 1g
Sugar alcohols: 0g
Protein: 14g

INGREDIENTS

3 cups shredded whole milk mozzarella cheese

5 ounces cream cheese, divided

2 cups almond flour

1 tablespoon baking powder

1½ teaspoons garlic powder

1½ teaspoons onion powder

2 large eggs

8 Applegate Naturals No Sugar Original Pork Breakfast Sausage links, cooked as directed and crumbled

1. Preheat oven to 400°F. Line a baking sheet with parchment paper and set aside.

2. Combine mozzarella cheese and 2 ounces cream cheese in a large microwave-safe bowl and microwave on high for 60 seconds. Remove from microwave, stir, and then heat for another 60 seconds or until melted.

3. Put melted cheeses in a food processor and add flour, baking powder, garlic powder, onion powder, and eggs. Pulse until a dough forms.

4. Place dough between two pieces of parchment paper and roll out to a 9" × 12" rectangle.

5. Combine remaining cream cheese and cooked sausage in a large bowl. Spread mixture evenly on prepared dough.

6. Starting at the 9" side, roll the dough into a tight log and seal by pinching the seams together. Cut dough into twelve equal-sized slices and transfer to prepared baking sheet.

7. Bake for 12 minutes or until top turns golden brown. Remove from oven and allow to cool for 5 minutes, then serve warm.

CHOCOLATE CHIP MUFFINS

Serves 12

Muffins aren't known for being the healthiest breakfast choice, but these keto-friendly Chocolate Chip Muffins pack healthy fats from the butter and loads of protein from the almond flour and eggs. If you don't have erythritol sweetener, you can substitute an equal amount of monk fruit sweetener in its place.

For half now

INGREDIENTS

¼ C

- 2½ cups almond flour
- ½ cup Swerve Brown sweetener *¼ C*
- 1 teaspoon baking powder *½ tsp*
- ¼ teaspoon sea salt *⅛ tsp*
- ⅓ cup salted grass-fed butter, softened *tbsp*
- ⅓ cup unsweetened almond milk
- 3 large eggs *1½ beaten divided*
- ¾ teaspoon vanilla extract
- ½ cup Lily's Milk Chocolate Style Baking Chips *¼ C*

1. Preheat oven to 350°F. Line a standard twelve-cup muffin tin with paper liners.

2. Combine flour, sweetener, baking powder, and salt in a large bowl. Set aside.

3. Place butter, almond milk, eggs, and vanilla in a separate large bowl and beat with a handheld electric mixer on low speed until fluffy, about 1 minute. Fold in flour mixture and mix until just combined. Stir in baking chips. Divide batter evenly among muffin cups.

4. Bake for 20 minutes or until a toothpick inserted in the center comes out clean.

5. Remove from oven and transfer muffins to a cooling rack. Allow to cool for 15 minutes, then serve warm.

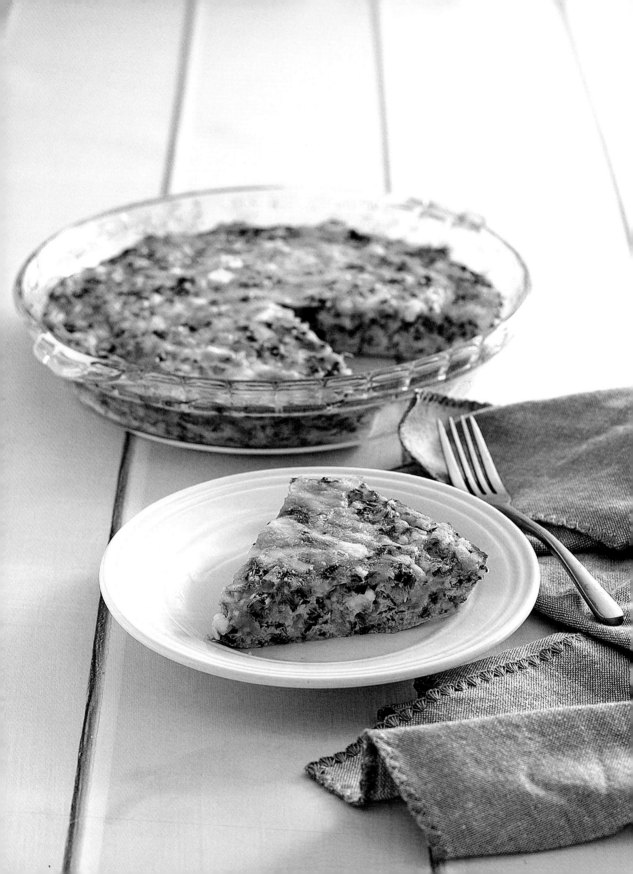

CHEESY SPINACH QUICHE

Serves 6

This quiche features spinach and feta for a traditional Greek flavor, but since eggs are so versatile, you can use this recipe as a base for whatever vegetables and cheeses you have on hand. It's a great, easy way to use up any leftover produce before it goes bad.

Calories: 319
Fat: 24g
Sodium: 718mg
Carbohydrates: 5g
Fiber: 2g
Sugar: 2g
Sugar alcohols: 0g
Protein: 21g

INGREDIENTS

1 tablespoon salted grass-fed butter

½ teaspoon minced garlic

1 medium shallot, peeled and minced

1 (10-ounce) package frozen chopped spinach, thawed and drained

6 large eggs, lightly beaten

2 cups shredded Monterey jack cheese

½ cup shredded Cheddar cheese

½ cup crumbled feta cheese

½ teaspoon sea salt

¼ teaspoon ground black pepper

1. Preheat oven to 350°F. Spray a 9" pie plate with cooking spray. Set aside.

2. Melt butter in a large skillet over medium-high heat. Add garlic and cook for 1 minute. Add shallot and cook for 3 more minutes. Stir in spinach and cook until heated through, about 3 minutes. Remove from heat.

3. Combine eggs, cheeses, salt, and pepper in a large bowl. Fold in spinach mixture and stir to incorporate. Transfer to prepared pie plate.

4. Bake for 30 minutes or until eggs have completely set. Remove from oven and allow to cool for 10 minutes, then serve warm.

CHICKEN SAUSAGE PATTIES

Serves 12

These patties are a delicious accompaniment to any keto breakfast. If you want to use them in a breakfast sandwich made with Everything Bagels (see recipe in this chapter), make sure to pat them down so they're thin enough to bite through.

(see recipe in this chapter)

NET CARBS

0g

Calories: 138
Fat: 8g
Sodium: 338mg
Carbohydrates: 3g
Fiber: 3g
Sugar: 0g
Sugar alcohols: 0g
Protein: 13g

INGREDIENTS

- 2 teaspoons ground sage
- 1½ teaspoons sea salt
- 1½ teaspoons garlic powder
- 1½ teaspoons onion powder
- 1 teaspoon ground black pepper
- 1 teaspoon dried parsley
- ¼ teaspoon crushed red pepper flakes
- ¼ teaspoon ground coriander
- 2 pounds ground chicken
- 2 tablespoons ChocZero Maple Syrup
- 2 tablespoons avocado oil

1. Combine sage, salt, garlic powder, onion powder, black pepper, parsley, red pepper flakes, and coriander in a large bowl and mix well.

2. Add ground chicken and maple syrup to bowl and use your hands to incorporate all ingredients evenly.

3. Divide mixture into twelve equal portions and form into patties.

4. Heat avocado oil in a large skillet over medium heat. Add sausage patties and cook for 5 minutes on each side or until chicken is no longer pink.

5. Remove from heat and serve.

JALAPEÑO CHEDDAR CHAFFLES

Serves 2 (Makes 4 [4"] chaffles)

These savory chaffles are delicious with just a little butter on top. You can also serve them with a side of eggs or use them as the bread for a sandwich—breakfast or otherwise.

Calories: 150
Fat: 11g
Sodium: 239mg
Carbohydrates: 2g
Fiber: 1g
Sugar: 1g
Sugar alcohols: 0g
Protein: 11g

INGREDIENTS

2 large egg whites

1 tablespoon almond flour

½ cup shredded Cheddar cheese

2 tablespoons diced fresh jalapeños

1. Preheat mini waffle maker.

2. Whisk egg whites in a medium bowl until light and fluffy. Stir in flour and cheese until combined. Fold in jalapeños.

3. Pour one-fourth of the batter into heated waffle maker. Cook for 3 minutes or until steam no longer comes out of waffle maker. Remove from waffle maker and repeat with remaining batter.

4. Serve immediately.

LEMON POPPYSEED MUG MUFFIN

Serves 1

With this mug muffin, you can have a yummy breakfast ready in minutes.

Calories: 171
Fat: 10g
Sodium: 374mg
Carbohydrates: 38g
Fiber: 4g
Sugar: 1g
Sugar alcohols: 30g
Protein: 9g

INGREDIENTS

1 tablespoon almond flour

1 tablespoon coconut flour

1 tablespoon Swerve Granular sweetener

¾ teaspoon baking powder

¾ teaspoon lemon extract

1 large egg, lightly beaten

1 tablespoon plus 1 teaspoon unsweetened almond milk, divided

¾ teaspoon poppy seeds

2 tablespoons Swerve Confectioners sweetener

1. Add dry ingredients to a 12-ounce microwave-safe mug. Stir to combine.

2. Stir in lemon extract, egg, and 1 tablespoon almond milk. Add poppy seeds.

3. Microwave for 60 seconds or until muffin sets and a toothpick inserted in center comes out clean.

4. Whisk confectioner's sweetener and remaining almond milk in a small bowl until smooth. Drizzle over muffin and serve immediately.

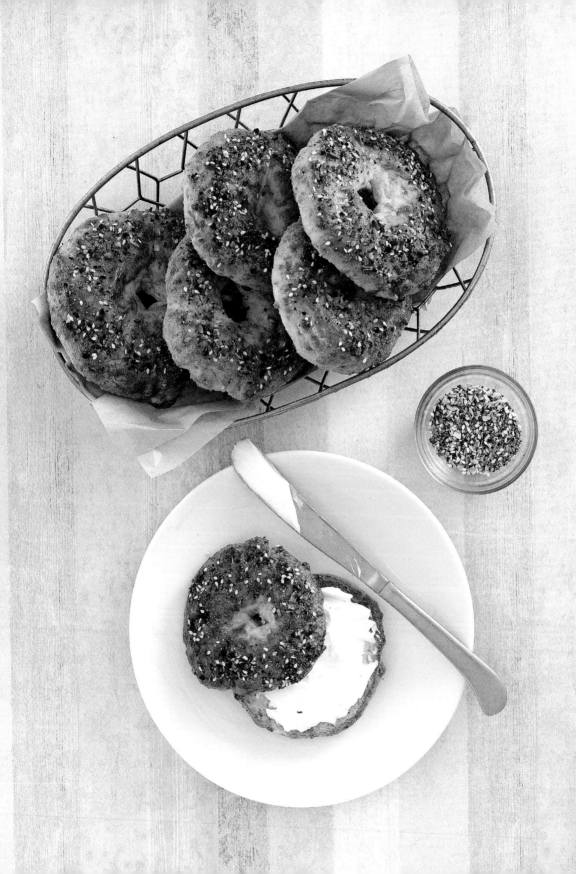

EVERYTHING BAGELS

Serves 6

These keto-friendly bagels taste even better than the "real" thing! After baking, you can toast them and spread some cream cheese on top or use them to make bacon, egg, and cheese breakfast sandwiches. They freeze well too, so you can double or triple the batch and save some for later.

NET CARBS
6g

Calories: 426
Fat: 34g
Sodium: 601mg
Carbohydrates: 10g
Fiber: 4g
Sugar: 2g
Sugar alcohols: 0g
Protein: 23g

INGREDIENTS

3 cups shredded whole milk mozzarella cheese

2 ounces cream cheese

2 cups almond flour

1 tablespoon baking powder

1½ teaspoons garlic powder

1½ teaspoons onion powder

3 large eggs, divided

2 tablespoons Trader Joe's Everything But the Bagel Sesame Seasoning Blend

1. Preheat oven to 425°F. Line a baking sheet with parchment paper and set aside.

2. Combine mozzarella cheese and cream cheese in a large microwave-safe bowl. Microwave on high for 90 seconds, stir, and then microwave for another 60 seconds or until melted. Transfer to a food processor.

3. Add flour, baking powder, garlic powder, onion powder, and 2 eggs to food processor. Pulse until a dough forms.

4. Divide dough into six portions and form each portion into a ball. Press your finger into the center of each ball to form a hole and make a ring. Arrange on prepared baking sheet, about 2 inches apart.

5. Lightly beat remaining egg and use a pastry brush to brush egg on top of each bagel. Sprinkle seasoning on top.

6. Bake for 12 minutes or until tops turn golden brown. Remove from oven and allow to cool for 5 minutes.

7. Slice in half and toast, if desired.

BACON CAULIFLOWER HASH

Serves 6

This Bacon Cauliflower Hash pairs perfectly with fried or scrambled eggs. If you want to make this recipe part of your weekly meal prep, hard-boil some eggs and you can easily take it all with you on the go.

INGREDIENTS

6 slices Applegate Naturals No Sugar Bacon

1 teaspoon minced garlic

1 medium yellow onion, peeled and diced

1 large head cauliflower, cut into florets

½ teaspoon paprika

1 teaspoon sea salt

½ teaspoon ground black pepper

3 tablespoons Kettle & Fire Classic Chicken Bone Broth

1 tablespoon chopped fresh parsley

1. Cook bacon in a large ungreased skillet over medium-high heat until crispy, about 4 minutes each side. Remove bacon from skillet and set on a paper towel–lined plate. Leave bacon fat in skillet and reduce heat to medium.

2. Add garlic and onion to skillet and cook until slightly softened, about 4 minutes. Add cauliflower and continue cooking for 3 minutes. Add paprika, salt, and pepper and stir to combine.

3. Pour in broth, reduce heat to low, and cover. Cook for 5 minutes until cauliflower is tender.

4. While cauliflower is cooking, roughly chop cooked bacon. Remove skillet from heat and stir in chopped bacon.

5. Sprinkle parsley on top and serve.

WATCH BACON INGREDIENTS

Most store-bought bacon has some form of sugar added to it. It may be brown sugar, maple syrup, or honey—none of which fit a keto diet. If you can't find no-sugar-added bacon at your local supermarket, you may be able to request it be made specifically from your local meat farmer or butcher shop.

OVERNIGHT MAPLE WALNUT N'OATMEAL

Serves 2

Instead of oats, which pack just over 13 grams of carbohydrates into ½ cup, this "n'oatmeal" uses hemp hearts. Not only are hemp hearts lower in carbs, but they contain lots of healthy fats too.

NET CARBS
4g

Calories: 351
Fat: 29g
Sodium: 152mg
Carbohydrates: 15g
Fiber: 11g
Sugar: 1g
Sugar alcohols: 0g
Protein: 16g

INGREDIENTS

⅔ cup unsweetened walnut milk

½ cup hemp hearts

1 tablespoon chia seeds

1 tablespoon ChocZero Maple Syrup

½ teaspoon vanilla extract

⅛ teaspoon sea salt

2 tablespoons crushed walnuts

1. Add all ingredients to a medium bowl and whisk to combine. Divide mixture in half between two 6-ounce Mason jars.

2. Cover and refrigerate overnight (or for at least 8 hours).

3. Remove from refrigerator and serve cold.

THE POWER OF HEMP

Hemp seeds are small, but they pack a lot of nutrition into that little package. More than 30 percent of the calories in hemp seeds comes from the fatty acids linoleic acid and alpha-linolenic acid, which help keep your heart healthy. Hemp seeds also contain about 25 percent high-quality protein, making them a great addition to a keto diet.

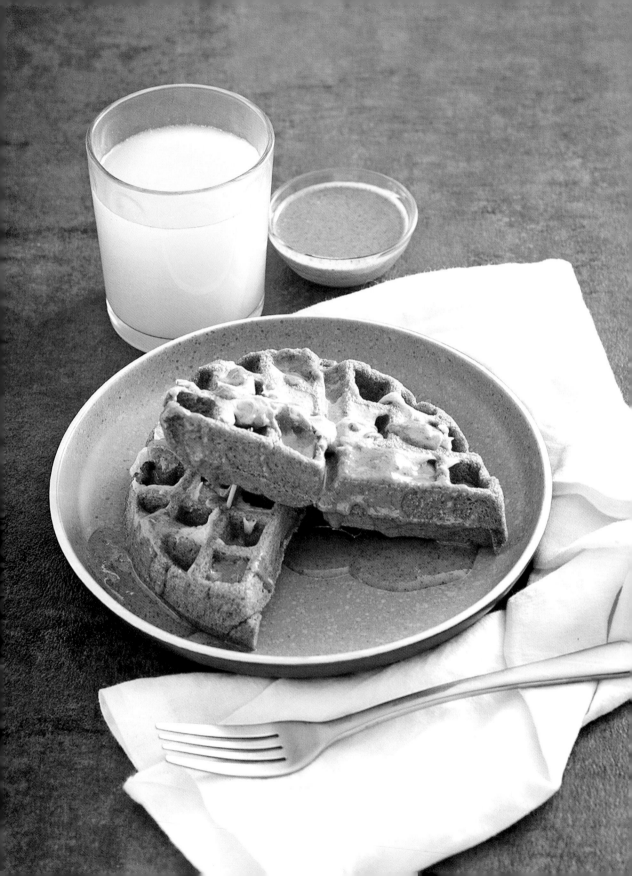

CINNAMON WAFFLES WITH CINNAMON CREAM CHEESE ICING

NET CARBS
4g

Calories: 301
Fat: 25g
Sodium: 206mg
Carbohydrates: 17g
Fiber: 3g
Sugar: 2g
Sugar alcohols: 10g
Protein: 12g

Serves 2

This decadent breakfast is a great choice on a slow weekend morning. In addition to the cream cheese icing, you can top these waffles with ChocZero Maple Syrup or some melted no-sugar-added almond butter.

INGREDIENTS

¼ cup plus 2 tablespoons almond flour

2 tablespoons Swerve Confectioners sweetener, divided

¼ teaspoon baking soda

1 teaspoon Perfect Keto Vanilla MCT Oil Powder

1 teaspoon ground cinnamon, divided

2 large eggs

1 teaspoon vanilla extract, divided

2 ounces cream cheese, softened

1. Preheat a standard waffle maker.

2. Combine flour, 1 tablespoon sweetener, baking soda, MCT oil powder, and ¾ teaspoon cinnamon in a medium bowl.

3. Whisk together eggs and ¾ teaspoon vanilla in a small bowl. Fold eggs into dry ingredients.

4. Pour batter into waffle maker and allow to cook according to waffle maker manufacturer directions.

5. While waffle is cooking, combine cream cheese, remaining sweetener, remaining cinnamon, and remaining vanilla in a separate small bowl, and beat until smooth.

6. Remove waffle from waffle maker and cut in half. Spread icing on top and serve immediately.

WHAT IS MCT OIL POWDER?

Medium-chain triglycerides (MCTs) are fatty acids that help stabilize blood sugar, increase production of ketones, reduce inflammation, boost metabolism, and improve brain function. They're found in high amounts in coconut products and palm oil. MCT oil powder is a supplemental form of MCT oil that gives you all the benefits of MCTs in a powdered form that's easy to incorporate into meals, fat bombs, and smoothies when you need to increase the healthy fat content.

MAPLE BACON MINI WAFFLES

Serves 2 (Makes 4 [4"] mini waffles)

Maple syrup and bacon make a dynamic flavor combination that you'll be going back to again and again. If you don't have a mini waffle maker, you can make these in a standard waffle maker, but you may want to double the batter and watch your portion size.

NET CARBS
3g

Calories: 322
Fat: 23g
Sodium: 584mg
Carbohydrates: 32g
Fiber: 28g
Sugar: 0g
Sugar alcohols: 1g
Protein: 12g

INGREDIENTS

2 large eggs

2 tablespoons Tessemae's Organic Mayonnaise

¼ teaspoon ground cinnamon

¼ teaspoon vanilla extract

½ teaspoon baking powder

½ teaspoon Swerve Granular sweetener

4 slices Applegate Naturals No Sugar Bacon, cooked and chopped

2 tablespoons salted grass-fed butter

¼ cup ChocZero Maple Syrup

1. Preheat a mini waffle maker.

2. Combine eggs, mayonnaise, cinnamon, vanilla, baking powder, and sweetener in a medium bowl, and whisk until combined. Fold in bacon.

3. Pour one-fourth of the batter into heated waffle maker. Cook for 3 minutes or until steam no longer comes out of waffle maker. Remove from waffle maker and repeat with remaining batter.

4. Top each waffle with equal amounts of butter and maple syrup and serve immediately.

CHAPTER 3

APPETIZERS AND SNACKS

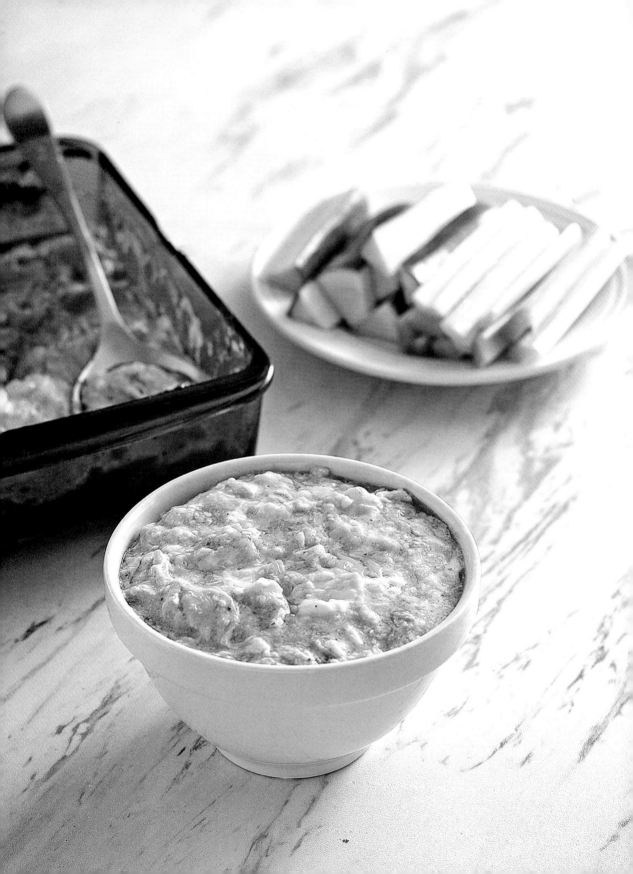

BUFFALO CHICKEN DIP

Serves 24 (¼ cup per serving)

The New Primal Medium Buffalo Sauce is a keto-friendly hot sauce with only 1 gram of net carbs per serving. Although it's categorized as "medium," this hot sauce does have a pretty good kick, so if you want to dial down the spice, opt for the mild version instead. Dip with celery sticks or raw zucchini slices!

INGREDIENTS

- 1 (12.5-ounce) can white chunk chicken breast, drained
- 1 cup The New Primal Medium Buffalo Sauce
- 2 (8-ounce) packages cream cheese, softened
- 1 cup Tessemae's Organic Creamy Ranch Dressing
- 2 cups shredded Cheddar cheese

1. Preheat oven to 350°F.

2. Combine chicken and buffalo sauce in a large bowl and toss to fully coat chicken. Transfer chicken to an ungreased 8" × 8" baking dish.

3. Add cream cheese and ranch dressing to a separate medium bowl and beat with a handheld electric mixer on medium speed until smooth. Pour mixture on top of chicken and spread evenly with a spatula.

4. Sprinkle Cheddar cheese on top of cream cheese mixture and bake for 30 minutes or until dip is hot and bubbly.

5. Remove from oven and allow to cool for 5 minutes, then serve warm.

CHICKEN PARMESAN DIP

Serves 12 (¼ cup per serving)

This dip is so good that you're going to want to eat it right from the dish with a spoon. Although that's certainly keto-friendly, you could also try scooping it with some raw zucchini slices, which have a crisp texture and mild taste.

Calories: 188
Fat: 15g
Sodium: 604mg
Carbohydrates: 3g
Fiber: 1g
Sugar: 1g
Sugar alcohols: 0g
Protein: 11g

INGREDIENTS

½ cup coarse almond meal

1 teaspoon Italian seasoning

2 tablespoons grated Parmesan cheese

1 (12.5-ounce) can white chunk chicken breast, drained

8 ounces cream cheese, softened

1 cup Rao's Homemade Marinara Sauce, divided

1 cup shredded whole milk mozzarella cheese

1. Preheat oven to 350°F.

2. Combine almond meal, Italian seasoning, and Parmesan cheese in a medium bowl. Add chicken and toss to coat.

3. Spread cream cheese in the bottom of an ungreased 8" × 8" baking dish. Spread ½ cup marinara sauce on cream cheese and top with chicken mixture.

4. Pour remaining sauce evenly over chicken and sprinkle mozzarella cheese on top.

5. Bake for 30 minutes or until hot and bubbly. Remove from oven and allow to cool for 5 minutes, then serve warm.

SAUSAGE AND CHEESE BITES

Serves 6 (Makes 18 bites)

These Sausage and Cheese Bites are a good go-to recipe when you're asked to bring an appetizer to a party but want to keep it keto. They're quick, easy, low in carbs, and (best of all) delicious enough to satisfy even the pickiest carb lover.

NET CARBS

0g

Calories: 331
Fat: 27g
Sodium: 568mg
Carbohydrates: 6g
Fiber: 3g
Sugar: 1g
Sugar alcohols: 3g
Protein: 19g

INGREDIENTS

1 pound no-sugar-added ground pork sausage

1 large egg, lightly beaten

1 teaspoon grass-fed heavy cream

½ cup Good Dee's Cracker Biscuit Mix

1 cup shredded Cheddar cheese

1 cup shredded pepper jack cheese

2 tablespoons minced yellow onion

¼ teaspoon garlic powder

1. Preheat oven to 350°F. Line a baking sheet with parchment paper and set aside.

2. Combine all ingredients in a large bowl and use your hands to incorporate everything together.

3. Form sausage mixture into eighteen 1" balls and arrange on prepared baking sheet.

4. Bake for 20 minutes or until browned and completely cooked through.

5. Remove from oven and allow to cool for 5 minutes, then serve warm.

SPICED ROASTED PUMPKIN SEEDS

Serves 6

Pumpkin seeds are the perfectly balanced keto snack. One serving (¼ cup) offers 14 grams of healthy fats with only 1 gram of net carbs. They're also rich in magnesium, a mineral that most Americans don't get nearly enough of.

Calories: 79
Fat: 6g
Sodium: 207mg
Carbohydrates: 2g
Fiber: 1g
Sugar: 0g
Sugar alcohols: 0g
Protein: 4g

INGREDIENTS

1½ cups raw whole pumpkin seeds

1 tablespoon unsalted grass-fed butter, melted

1 teaspoon chili powder

½ teaspoon sea salt

½ teaspoon garlic salt

¼ teaspoon cayenne pepper

1. Preheat oven to 350°F. Line two baking sheets with parchment paper and set aside.

2. Combine pumpkin seeds and melted butter in a medium bowl and toss to coat.

3. Mix chili powder, sea salt, garlic salt, and cayenne pepper in a separate small bowl, and sprinkle over pumpkin seeds. Toss to coat evenly.

4. Spread pumpkin seeds in a single layer on prepared baking sheets.

5. Bake for 20 minutes. Remove from oven and stir, then rearrange in a single layer. Bake for another 20 minutes or until golden brown.

6. Remove from oven and allow to cool for 5 minutes, then serve warm.

MEET YOUR MAGNESIUM NEEDS

Magnesium is connected to more than three hundred chemical reactions in your body. It keeps your muscles and bones healthy and helps calm your nervous system, among other things. A 2018 report in Open Heart *(a cardiology journal) calls magnesium deficiency "a public health crisis" that's one of the leading causes of chronic diseases like heart disease. A ¼-cup serving of pumpkin seeds can help you meet your needs by supplying almost half of the magnesium that you need for the entire day.*

PIZZA BITES

Serves 6 (Makes 24 bites)

You won't even miss the crust when you try these Pizza Bites. And the best part? You can make them in under 5 minutes. The pepperoni gives each bite structure *and* a pop of flavor.

NET CARBS
1g

Calories: 88
Fat: 8g
Sodium: 231mg
Carbohydrates: 1g
Fiber: 0g
Sugar: 1g
Sugar alcohols: 0g
Protein: 4g

INGREDIENTS

24 slices no-sugar-added pepperoni

½ cup Rao's Homemade Marinara Sauce

½ cup shredded whole milk mozzarella cheese

1. Position oven rack in the middle of the oven. Preheat broiler on high. Line a baking sheet with parchment paper. Line a second baking sheet with paper towels. Set both aside.

2. Arrange pepperoni slices in a single layer on parchment-lined baking sheet.

3. Put 1 teaspoon marinara sauce on each pepperoni slice and spread out with a spoon. Add 1 teaspoon cheese on top of marinara.

4. Put the baking sheet in the oven and broil for 3 minutes or until cheese is melted and slightly browned.

5. Remove from oven and transfer bites to paper towel–lined baking sheet to absorb excess grease. Allow to cool for 5 minutes, then serve warm.

MAPLE-ROASTED ALMONDS

Serves 8 (¼ cup per serving)

While many keto sweeteners fall short, ChocZero Maple Syrup has both the thickness and flavor of the real thing, but with only 1 gram of net carbs per serving and no preservatives. This recipe calls for the original flavor, but you can also try it with the Maple Vanilla or Maple Pecan varieties.

INGREDIENTS

2 cups shelled whole raw almonds

⅓ cup ChocZero Maple Syrup

3 tablespoons Swerve Granular sweetener

1 teaspoon ground cinnamon

1. Preheat oven to 350°F. Line a baking sheet with parchment paper. Line a second baking sheet with paper towels. Set both aside.

2. Place almonds in a medium bowl. In a separate small bowl, combine maple syrup, sweetener, and cinnamon and mix well.

3. Pour mixture over almonds and toss to coat.

4. Transfer almonds to parchment-lined baking sheet and arrange in a single layer.

5. Bake for 15 minutes, stir and flip nuts, and then bake for another 15 minutes, watching the almonds carefully so they don't burn.

6. Remove from oven and allow to cool for 5 minutes. Scrape nuts off of pan and transfer to paper towel–lined baking sheet. Allow to cool completely before serving or placing in a bowl or container.

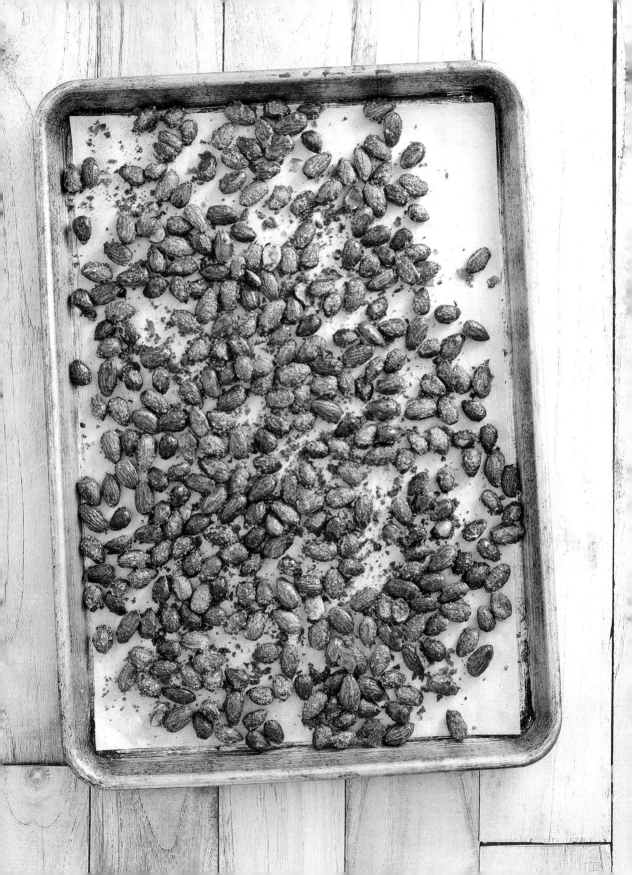

FRIED PICKLES

Serves 6

For a fully satisfying appetizer or snack, serve these Fried Pickles with a side of Tessemae's Organic Habanero Ranch Dressing. It adds a little kick that's similar to the dipping sauce you get alongside fried pickles at a restaurant. If you don't have an air fryer, you can pan-fry these in avocado oil, but note that this will affect the nutritional information.

NET CARBS

2g

Calories: 297
Fat: 21g
Sodium: 969mg
Carbohydrates: 4g
Fiber: 2g
Sugar: 2g
Sugar alcohols: 0g
Protein: 23g

INGREDIENTS

2 large eggs

¾ cup grass-fed heavy cream

¼ teaspoon cayenne pepper

2 cups crushed EPIC Oven Baked Pink Himalayan and Sea Salt Pork Rinds

½ cup almond flour

2 teaspoons paprika

1½ teaspoons ground black pepper

½ teaspoon sea salt

36 slices Woodstock Organic Kosher Dill Pickles

1. Preheat air fryer to 400°F.

2. Combine eggs, cream, and cayenne pepper in a large bowl, and whisk until combined.

3. Add pork rinds to a food processor and pulse until coarse crumbs form.

4. Add flour, paprika, black pepper, and salt to the food processor, and pulse until combined.

5. Transfer pork rind mixture to a shallow dish.

6. Coat each pickle chip with pork rind mixture, dip in egg mixture, then coat with pork rind mixture again.

7. Arrange coated pickle slices in a single layer in the air fryer basket (working in batches if necessary). Cook for 5 minutes, turn slices over, then cook for another 5 minutes or until golden brown.

8. Remove from air fryer and repeat with remaining pickle slices.

9. Allow to cool for 5 minutes, then serve warm.

BLT DIP

Serves 12 (¼ cup per serving)

If you want to make this a true BLT dip, sprinkle some chopped lettuce on top after the dip finishes baking. Serve with raw sliced zucchini or cucumber coins.

INGREDIENTS

½ cup Tessemae's Organic Mayonnaise

½ cup sour cream

8 ounces cream cheese, softened

2 cups shredded Cheddar cheese

1 large beefsteak tomato, seeded and diced

1 (12-ounce) package Applegate Naturals No Sugar Bacon, cooked and crumbled

1 tablespoon chopped green onions

1. Preheat oven to 350°F.

2. Combine mayonnaise, sour cream, and cream cheese in a large bowl, and beat with a handheld electric mixer on medium speed until smooth. Beat in Cheddar cheese.

3. Stir in tomato, bacon, and green onions.

4. Transfer mixture to an ungreased 8" × 8" baking dish and bake for 20 minutes or until dip is hot and bubbly.

5. Remove from oven and allow to cool for 5 minutes, then serve warm.

CHEESY TACO DIP

Serves 24 (¼ cup per serving)

This Cheesy Taco Dip is the perfect keto substitute for shelled tacos next time Taco Tuesday comes around. Serve it with raw zucchini slices, which add a nice crunch. The flavor is so mild that you won't even know you're eating zucchini.

NET CARBS
3g

Calories: 164
Fat: 14g
Sodium: 202mg
Carbohydrates: 4g
Fiber: 1g
Sugar: 2g
Sugar alcohols: 0g
Protein: 7g

INGREDIENTS

1 tablespoon chili powder

1½ teaspoons ground cumin

1 teaspoon sea salt

1 teaspoon ground black pepper

½ teaspoon paprika

¼ teaspoon garlic powder

¼ teaspoon onion powder

¼ teaspoon dried oregano

¼ teaspoon crushed red pepper flakes

1 tablespoon olive oil

1 pound 85/15 ground beef

1 (16-ounce) container sour cream

1 (8-ounce) package cream cheese, softened

1 (16-ounce) jar no-sugar-added salsa

1 small green bell pepper, seeded and finely chopped

1 (6-ounce) can sliced black olives, drained

2 cups shredded Cheddar cheese

1. Preheat oven to 350°F.

2. Combine spices in a small bowl and mix well. Set aside.

3. Heat olive oil in a large skillet over medium heat. Crumble ground beef into skillet and cook for 3 minutes. Sprinkle spices on beef and continue cooking until browned, about 5 more minutes. Remove from heat and set aside.

4. Combine sour cream and cream cheese in a large bowl and beat with a handheld electric mixer on medium speed until smooth.

5. Spread cream cheese mixture in the bottom of an ungreased 8" × 8" baking dish. Scoop beef onto cream cheese mixture and spread evenly.

6. Spread salsa evenly over the beef, then layer with bell pepper, then olives. Sprinkle Cheddar cheese evenly on top.

7. Bake for 30 minutes or until hot and bubbly. Remove from oven and allow to cool for 5 minutes, then serve warm.

MOZZARELLA STICKS

Serves 6

Make sure you arrange these mozzarella sticks in a single layer when cooking. Otherwise, they may stick together. If you don't have an air fryer, you can bake them at 350°F for about 20 minutes or until the coating turns golden brown.

NET CARBS

6g

Calories: 343
Fat: 25g
Sodium: 414mg
Carbohydrates: 9g
Fiber: 3g
Sugar: 2g
Sugar alcohols: 0g
Protein: 22g

INGREDIENTS

1½ cups coarse almond meal

1 teaspoon Italian seasoning

½ teaspoon garlic powder

½ teaspoon onion powder

½ teaspoon dried parsley

3 large eggs

12 (1-ounce) sticks mozzarella string cheese

1. Preheat air fryer to 400°F.

2. Combine almond meal, Italian seasoning, garlic powder, onion powder, and parsley in a shallow dish. Add eggs to a separate medium bowl and whisk lightly.

3. Cut each cheese stick in half crosswise.

4. Dip each cheese stick in eggs and then in almond meal mixture, coating evenly.

5. Arrange coated cheese sticks in a single layer in the air fryer basket. (You may need to cook cheese sticks in batches.) Cook for 6 minutes. Flip cheese sticks over and cook for another 6 minutes or until golden brown.

6. Remove from air fryer and repeat with remaining cheese sticks if necessary.

7. Remove from air fryer. Allow to cool for 5 minutes, then serve warm.

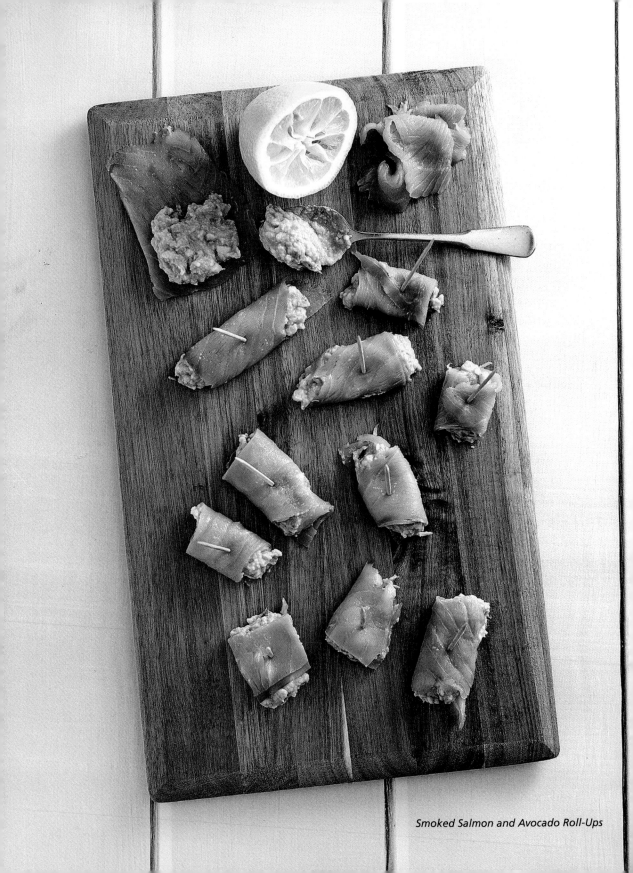

Smoked Salmon and Avocado Roll-Ups

SMOKED SALMON AND AVOCADO ROLL-UPS

Serves 1

NET CARBS 2g

Calories: 261
Fat: 18g
Sodium: 869mg
Carbohydrates: 9g
Fiber: 7g
Sugar: 1g
Sugar alcohols: 0g
Protein: 18g

These roll-ups make a delicious party food or an easy appetizer. They're also a great dairy-free fat bomb on those days when you're looking for a savory option.

INGREDIENTS

½ medium avocado, peeled and pitted

1 teaspoon fresh lemon juice

⅛ teaspoon sea salt

3 (1-ounce) slices smoked salmon

1. In a small bowl, combine avocado, lemon juice, and salt. Mash with a fork.

2. Spread one-third of the avocado mixture evenly on top of each salmon slice. Roll slices into individual rolls and secure with a toothpick.

3. Serve immediately.

CHILE CON QUESO

Serves 6 (3 tablespoons per serving)

NET CARBS 1g

Calories: 220
Fat: 19g
Sodium: 695mg
Carbohydrates: 1g
Fiber: 0g
Sugar: 0g
Sugar alcohols: 0g
Protein: 12g

This Chile con Queso rivals the appetizer you'd find at your favorite Mexican restaurant, but with considerably fewer carbs and only a handful of ingredients. Because it doesn't contain any emulsifiers, it will thicken up as it cools, but you can simply put it in the microwave or back on the stove for a few seconds to get it melted and smooth again.

INGREDIENTS

¼ cup grass-fed heavy cream

10 ounces Applegate Organics American Cheese, cut into smaller pieces

1 (4.5-ounce) can chopped green chiles

½ teaspoon ground cumin

½ teaspoon garlic salt

1. Combine cream and cheese in a medium saucepan over medium-low heat. Heat, stirring frequently, until cheese is melted and mixture is smooth.

2. Stir in chiles. Add cumin and garlic salt and stir to combine.

3. Remove from heat and serve immediately.

BAKED CHICKEN WINGS

NET CARBS
3g

Calories: 699
Fat: 52g
Sodium: 889mg
Carbohydrates: 4g
Fiber: 1g
Sugar: 0g
Sugar alcohols: 0g
Protein: 52g

Serves 4

Chicken wings are a party favorite, and with this recipe, you can easily make a batch in your oven instead of standing over a deep fryer and missing out on the fun. If you're serving a crowd, simply double or triple the recipe and rotate the racks in the oven every 20 minutes or so to make sure they're all evenly cooked.

INGREDIENTS

¼ cup olive oil

2 teaspoons minced garlic

1 tablespoon chili powder

1 tablespoon garlic powder

1 teaspoon onion powder

1 teaspoon sea salt

½ teaspoon ground black pepper

24 bone-in, skin-on chicken wings

1. Preheat oven to 375°F. Line a baking sheet with parchment paper and set aside.

2. Combine olive oil, minced garlic, chili powder, garlic powder, onion powder, salt, and pepper in a large bowl, and whisk until evenly incorporated.

3. Add chicken wings to bowl and toss to coat.

4. Spread chicken wings on prepared baking sheet and bake for 1 hour or until chicken is no longer pink and outside skins are crispy.

5. Remove from oven and serve immediately.

BACON AND CHIVE–STUFFED TOMATOES

Serves 6

If you're having trouble getting the tomatoes to stand up-right, slice a little off of the bottom to create a flat surface. When the tomatoes are sturdy, you can stuff them more easily. You can use cocktail tomatoes or large-sized cherry tomatoes.

INGREDIENTS

24 large cherry tomatoes

1 teaspoon sea salt

¼ cup Tessemae's Organic Mayonnaise

2 ounces cream cheese, softened

1 pound Applegate Naturals No Sugar Bacon, cooked and crumbled

¼ cup chopped fresh chives

¼ cup shredded Cheddar cheese

¼ teaspoon garlic powder

¼ teaspoon onion powder

1. Cut tops off each tomato and scoop out the insides with a small spoon. Discard.

2. Sprinkle salt into each tomato and turn them upside down on a paper towel. Allow to sit for 10 minutes or until excess juices drain from tomatoes.

3. Combine mayonnaise and cream cheese in a large bowl and beat with a handheld electric mixer on medium speed until smooth. Add remaining ingredients and stir until incorporated.

4. Scoop mixture evenly into tomatoes. Refrigerate for 2 hours before serving.

CHEESY RANCH CAULIFLOWER BITES

Serves 6 (Makes 24 bites)

Ranch-inspired seasoning is a zesty complement to cauliflower in these "no-tater" tot, low-carbohydrate cauliflower bites. For a spicy treat, dip them in buffalo sauce before eating.

NET CARBS
4g

Calories: 107
Fat: 6g
Sodium: 628mg
Carbohydrates: 6g
Fiber: 2g
Sugar: 2g
Sugar alcohols: 0g
Protein: 8g

INGREDIENTS

1 large head cauliflower, cut into florets

2 large eggs, lightly beaten

1¼ cups shredded Cheddar cheese, divided

1 tablespoon dried parsley

1 teaspoon dried dill

1 teaspoon garlic powder

1 teaspoon onion powder

1 teaspoon sea salt

½ teaspoon ground black pepper

6 slices Applegate Naturals No Sugar Bacon, cooked and crumbled

2 teaspoons dried chives

1. Preheat oven to 375°F. Grease cups of a twenty-four-cup mini muffin tin with olive oil cooking spray. Set aside.

2. Place cauliflower florets in a food processor and pulse until large crumbles form.

3. Transfer cauliflower to a fine-mesh cheesecloth and squeeze excess moisture out. Place cauliflower in a large bowl and add eggs, 1 cup cheese, seasonings, bacon, and chives. Mix well.

4. Fill each muffin cup with equal amounts of cauliflower mixture and top with remaining cheese.

5. Bake for 20 minutes or until golden brown. Remove from oven and allow to cool for 5 minutes, then serve warm.

SAVORY HERB CHAFFLES

Serves 2 (Makes 4 [4"] chaffles)

These Savory Herb Chaffles are excellent with a simple topping of grass-fed butter or herbed cream cheese. If you want to crisp them up, you can toast them a little bit after they come out of the waffle maker.

INGREDIENTS

2 large eggs

2 ounces cream cheese, softened

1 tablespoon coconut flour

¾ teaspoon Italian seasoning

½ teaspoon minced garlic

¼ teaspoon onion powder

¼ teaspoon sea salt

1 cup shredded whole milk mozzarella cheese, divided

1. Preheat a mini waffle maker.

2. Combine eggs, cream cheese, coconut flour, Italian seasoning, garlic, onion powder, and salt in a medium bowl, and beat with a handheld electric mixer on medium speed until smooth.

3. Sprinkle 2 tablespoons mozzarella cheese evenly on waffle maker. Allow to melt and then pour one-fourth of the batter on top. Sprinkle another 2 tablespoons mozzarella cheese on top.

4. Close waffle maker and cook for 3 minutes or until steam no longer comes out of waffle maker. Remove from waffle maker and repeat with remaining batter.

5. Serve immediately.

ZUCCHINI CHIPS

Serves 4

Pork rinds are an ideal keto substitute for breading because they add a crunch that's hard to achieve with almond flour alone, and each serving provides 4.5 grams of fat, 8 grams of protein, and absolutely no carbs.

INGREDIENTS

1 cup crushed EPIC Oven Baked Pink Himalayan and Sea Salt Pork Rinds

¾ cup grated Parmesan cheese

½ teaspoon sea salt

¼ teaspoon ground black pepper

1 large egg

1 medium zucchini, sliced into thin coins

¼ cup unsalted grass-fed butter, melted

1. Preheat air fryer to 350°F.

2. Combine pork rinds, cheese, salt, and pepper in a shallow dish and mix well.

3. Break egg into a small bowl and whisk lightly.

4. Dip zucchini slices in egg and then press into pork rind mixture, coating both sides evenly. Drizzle butter on top.

5. Arrange zucchini in a single layer in the air fryer basket. (You may need to cook them in batches.) Cook for 7 minutes, turn each zucchini slice over, and then cook for another 5 minutes.

6. Remove from air fryer and repeat with remaining zucchini if necessary. Allow to cool for 5 minutes, then serve warm.

BUFFALO CHICKEN CELERY BOATS

Serves 6

These celery boats are best served with Tessemae's Organic Creamy Ranch Dressing or your own homemade, keto-friendly ranch or blue cheese dressing. If you're not serving all of them at once, keep the celery crisp by waiting to fill it until right before you're ready to eat.

NET CARBS
2g

Calories: 146
Fat: 6g
Sodium: 744mg
Carbohydrates: 3g
Fiber: 1g
Sugar: 1g
Sugar alcohols: 0g
Protein: 18g

INGREDIENTS

2 cups canned white chunk chicken breast, drained

3 tablespoons Tessemae's Organic Mayonnaise

¼ cup Frank's RedHot Original Cayenne Pepper Sauce

¼ teaspoon sea salt

⅛ teaspoon ground black pepper

12 medium stalks celery, cut into 4" pieces

1. Combine chicken, mayonnaise, pepper sauce, salt, and pepper in a medium mixing bowl.

2. Scoop mixture evenly into wells of celery stalks.

3. Serve immediately.

THE POWER OF CELERY

Celery is a nutrient powerhouse. It's anti-inflammatory, anti-hypertensive (which means it can help keep blood pressure normal), and full of antioxidants. Celery is also rich in dietary fiber, which can help boost weight loss and contribute to healthy digestion. And since about half of the carbohydrates in celery come from fiber, the net carb count is low, making them a very keto-friendly choice.

CRUNCHY CHEESY CHAFFLES

Serves 2 (Makes 4 [4"] chaffles)

Kerrygold Dubliner is a grass-fed cheese that tastes like a mixture of Cheddar, Swiss, and Parmesan all rolled into one. It's a great choice for chaffles, not only because of its unique flavor, but also because it melts really evenly and smoothly.

INGREDIENTS

4 large eggs

1 cup shredded Cheddar cheese

2 tablespoons crushed EPIC Oven Baked Pink Himalayan and Sea Salt Pork Rinds

2 teaspoons nutritional yeast

½ cup shredded Kerrygold Dubliner cheese, divided

1. Preheat a mini waffle maker.

2. Combine eggs, Cheddar cheese, pork rinds, and nutritional yeast in a large bowl, and whisk until evenly incorporated.

3. Sprinkle 1 tablespoon Dubliner cheese evenly on preheated waffle maker. Pour one-fourth of the batter on top. Sprinkle another 1 tablespoon Dubliner cheese on top.

4. Close waffle maker and cook for 3 minutes or until steam no longer comes out of waffle maker. Remove from waffle maker and repeat with remaining batter.

5. Serve immediately.

SPICY PIMENTO CHEESE DIP

NET CARBS
2g

Calories: 153
Fat: 14g
Sodium: 249mg
Carbohydrates: 2g
Fiber: 0g
Sugar: 1g
Sugar alcohols: 0g
Protein: 6g

Serves 12 (¼ cup per serving)

Pimento peppers, also called cherry peppers, are a mildly spicy, mostly sweet variety of pepper that complements the sharp flavor of the Cheddar cheese in this recipe perfectly. If you're using jarred or canned pimento peppers instead of fresh ones, read the ingredient list carefully to make sure there's no added sugar. Serve with raw zucchini slices.

INGREDIENTS

8 ounces cream cheese, softened

2 cups shredded Cheddar cheese

½ cup Tessemae's Organic Mayonnaise

1 teaspoon Frank's RedHot Original Cayenne Pepper Sauce

½ cup seeded and diced pimento peppers

½ teaspoon garlic powder

½ teaspoon onion powder

½ teaspoon cayenne pepper

¼ teaspoon dry mustard

¼ teaspoon sea salt

¼ teaspoon ground black pepper

Combine all ingredients in a large bowl and beat with a handheld electric mixer on medium speed until combined. Serve immediately.

SMOKED SALMON DEVILED EGGS

Serves 6

NET CARBS
2g

Calories: 287
Fat: 19g
Sodium: 705mg
Carbohydrates: 4g
Fiber: 2g
Sugar: 1g
Sugar alcohols: 0g
Protein: 24g

These Smoked Salmon Deviled Eggs combine omega-3 fatty acids from the salmon and monounsaturated fats from the avocado with high-quality protein from the eggs. It's a perfectly balanced keto appetizer or snack that you can easily take with you on the go.

INGREDIENTS

12 large eggs, hard-boiled

1 tablespoon Frank's RedHot Original Cayenne Pepper Sauce

¾ cup Tessemae's Organic Mayonnaise

¼ teaspoon sea salt

2 tablespoons chopped fresh dill

12 (1-ounce) strips smoked salmon

1 medium avocado, peeled, pitted, and cut into 24 slices

1. Cut hard-boiled eggs in half and transfer yolks to a small bowl. Mash yolks with a fork and add pepper sauce, mayonnaise, salt, and dill. Continue mashing until combined.

2. Scoop yolk mixture into egg whites.

3. Cut salmon strips in half and top each prepared egg half with a piece of salmon and a slice of avocado.

4. Serve immediately.

CHAPTER 4

SOUPS
AND SALADS

CREAMY CHICKEN AND BACON SOUP

Serves 6

Bacon is a keto dieter's best friend, but many commercial varieties have added sugar. Applegate Naturals has a delicious, no-sugar-added option that's becoming increasingly available in many commercial grocery stores. If you're having difficulty finding it, visit www.applegate.com and use the Where to Buy search engine.

NET CARBS
4g

Calories: 576
Fat: 49g
Sodium: 1,211mg
Carbohydrates: 5g
Fiber: 1g
Sugar: 3g
Sugar alcohols: 0g
Protein: 30g

INGREDIENTS

6 slices Applegate Naturals No Sugar Bacon, chopped

1 medium shallot, peeled and diced

1 teaspoon minced garlic

1 medium stalk celery, finely diced

4 cups Kettle & Fire Classic Chicken Bone Broth

12 ounces boneless, skinless chicken breasts, cooked and shredded

1 teaspoon sea salt

½ teaspoon ground black pepper

½ cup salted grass-fed butter

2 teaspoons xanthan gum

2 cups grass-fed heavy cream

1. Add bacon to a large stockpot and cook over medium heat until browned, about 7 minutes. Add shallot and cook for another 2 minutes or until softened.

2. Stir in garlic and cook for 30 seconds. Add celery and continue cooking for 4 more minutes.

3. Add broth, chicken breasts, salt, and pepper, and reduce heat to low. Simmer for 1 hour.

4. Heat butter in a small saucepan over medium heat. Once melted, add xanthan gum and whisk until smooth, about 1 minute.

5. Slowly whisk in cream. Reduce heat to medium-low and cook until thickened, about 5 minutes, whisking frequently.

6. Stir cream mixture into soup and simmer for another 30 minutes.

7. Remove from heat. Allow to cool for 5 minutes, then serve warm.

BUFFALO CHICKEN COBB SALAD

Serves 4

If you prefer not to use canned chicken, you can certainly cook your own chicken breasts or thighs for this salad. Another convenient option is to pick up a rotisserie chicken from the deli. Just make sure you're reading ingredient lists and choosing one that doesn't have added sugar (many do).

NET CARBS

6g

Calories: 524
Fat: 39g
Sodium: 1,382mg
Carbohydrates: 10g
Fiber: 4g
Sugar: 3g
Sugar alcohols: 0g
Protein: 33g

INGREDIENTS

1 (12.5-ounce) can white chunk chicken breast, drained

¼ cup The New Primal Medium Buffalo Sauce

4 cups romaine lettuce

4 large eggs, hard-boiled and chopped

1 medium avocado, peeled, pitted, and chopped

¼ cup chopped black olives

4 slices Applegate Naturals No Sugar Bacon, cooked and crumbled

¼ cup shredded Cheddar cheese

½ cup Tessemae's Organic Habanero Ranch Dressing

1. Place chicken and buffalo sauce in a medium bowl and toss to combine. Set aside.

2. Place 1 cup lettuce on each of four plates. Top each plate with one-fourth of the chopped eggs, one-fourth of the avocado, 1 tablespoon olives, 1 tablespoon crumbled bacon, and 1 tablespoon cheese.

3. Scoop equal amounts of chicken mixture on top of each salad.

4. Drizzle 2 tablespoons dressing evenly over each salad and serve immediately.

SAUERKRAUT AND BACON BISQUE

Serves 6

You don't have to use Cleveland Kraut sauerkraut for this recipe (although it's a delicious and high-quality choice), but if you're using a different brand, try to find one that's raw and probiotic-rich instead of highly processed.

NET CARBS
5g

Calories: 994
Fat: 84g
Sodium: 2,957mg
Carbohydrates: 7g
Fiber: 2g
Sugar: 5g
Sugar alcohols: 0g
Protein: 53g

INGREDIENTS

24 ounces (2 packages) Applegate Naturals No Sugar Bacon

1 medium yellow onion, peeled and finely chopped

1 teaspoon xanthan gum

3 cups grass-fed heavy cream

1½ cups Cleveland Kraut Roasted Garlic sauerkraut

1 tablespoon minced fresh thyme

½ teaspoon sea salt

¼ teaspoon ground black pepper

1 tablespoon fresh lemon juice

1. Add bacon to a large stockpot and cook over medium heat until browned and crispy, about 7 minutes. Add onion and cook until softened, about 3 minutes.

2. Stir in xanthan gum and then pour in cream. Reduce heat to medium-low and cook until thickened, stirring frequently, about 10 minutes.

3. Add sauerkraut, thyme, salt, and pepper, and stir to combine. Cook for 2 minutes and then stir in lemon juice.

4. Remove from heat and serve immediately.

PROBIOTICS IN SAUERKRAUT

There's a lot of focus on taking probiotic supplements for gut health, but fermented vegetables like sauerkraut are actually one of the richest (and most bioavailable) sources. A 2-tablespoon serving of sauerkraut contains around 1 million colony-forming units (or CFUs), which is enough to give you all the probiotics that you need for the day. As an added bonus, sauerkraut also contains a wider variety of bacterial strains than supplements, and those bacteria can survive the passage through your stomach acid better than the bacteria in supplements.

KALE AND AVOCADO SALAD

Serves 4

Massaging the kale with the oil and lemon mixture before preparing the rest of the salad softens the leaves so that they're not as tough as they are fully raw. If you're still not a fan of the texture, you can use baby kale, which is milder and less tough.

INGREDIENTS

¼ cup olive oil

2 tablespoons fresh lemon juice

2 tablespoons Dijon mustard

½ teaspoon sea salt

¼ teaspoon ground black pepper

4 cups chopped fresh kale

1 small avocado, peeled, pitted, and diced

½ cup chopped cucumber

¼ cup chopped red bell pepper

2 tablespoons chopped red onion

2 tablespoons crumbled blue cheese

1. Combine olive oil, lemon juice, mustard, salt, and black pepper in a small bowl, and whisk to combine.

2. Put kale in a separate large bowl and add dressing. Use your hands to massage the dressing into the leaves. Allow the mixture to sit for 5 minutes.

3. Add remaining ingredients and toss to combine. Serve immediately.

CREAM OF MUSHROOM SOUP

Serves 6

Many throw-together and easy casserole recipes call for cream of mushroom soup, but the kind you find in a can at the store is not suitable for a keto diet. You can use this low-carb cream of mushroom soup in place of the store-bought kind in any recipe or just eat it on its own. If you want to have it on hand for when a recipe calls for it, make extra and freeze it in cup-sized servings.

INGREDIENTS

4 tablespoons salted grass-fed butter, divided

1 small yellow onion, peeled and finely diced

5 cups sliced baby bella mushrooms

½ teaspoon sea salt

¼ teaspoon dried thyme

1½ cups Kettle & Fire Classic Chicken Bone Broth

½ teaspoon xanthan gum

¼ teaspoon ground black pepper

1 cup grass-fed heavy cream

1. Heat 1 tablespoon butter in a large stockpot over medium heat. Add onion and cook until softened, about 3 minutes. Add mushrooms, salt, and thyme, and cook for another 5 minutes.

2. Stir in bone broth and reduce heat to low. Simmer for 15 minutes.

3. Transfer to a blender (you may have to work in batches) and purée until mixture is mostly smooth but still has some chunks.

4. Heat remaining butter in stockpot. Stir in xanthan gum.

5. Add mushroom purée, pepper, and cream, and stir until smooth. Simmer for 5 minutes, stirring constantly.

6. Remove from heat and serve.

CURRIED SAUERKRAUT SALAD

Serves 6

You can make this recipe with any sauerkraut, but the Cleveland Kraut is a top-of-the-line choice that's made with high-quality ingredients and no added sugar. If you can only find plain kraut, just add a teaspoon of curry powder when you're tossing ingredients together.

NET CARBS
3g

Calories: 118
Fat: 10g
Sodium: 553mg
Carbohydrates: 12g
Fiber: 3g
Sugar: 3g
Sugar alcohols: 6g
Protein: 1g

INGREDIENTS

¼ cup avocado oil

½ cup apple cider vinegar

¼ cup Swerve Confectioners sweetener

4 cups Cleveland Kraut Curry Kraut sauerkraut

1 small yellow onion, peeled and finely diced

1 medium stalk celery, finely diced

¼ cup chopped red bell pepper

1. Combine oil, vinegar, and sweetener in a small saucepan over low heat and stir until sweetener is incorporated into mixture. Remove from heat and allow to cool to room temperature.

2. Add remaining ingredients to a large bowl and toss to combine. Pour oil mixture on top and toss again to coat.

3. Refrigerate for 2 hours before serving.

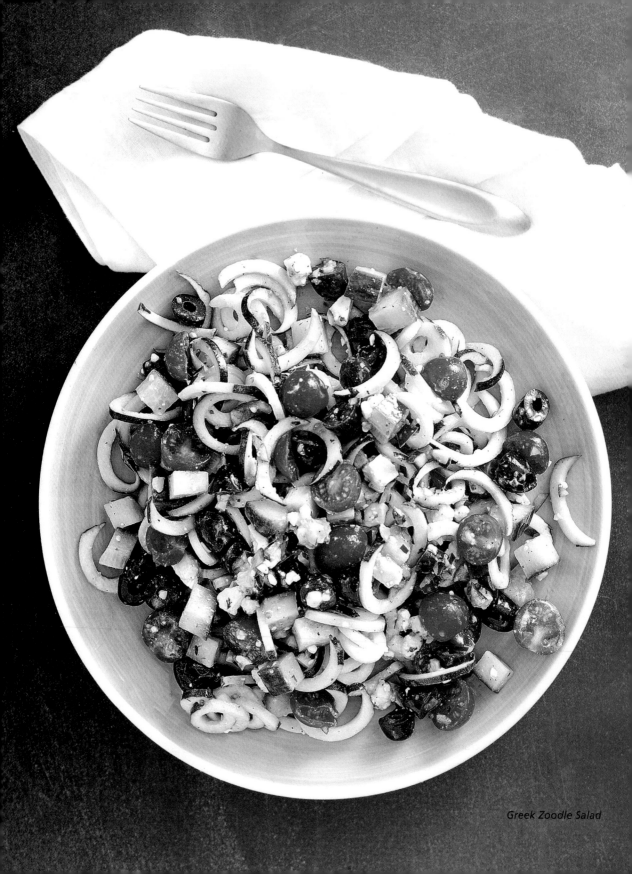

Greek Zoodle Salad

GREEK ZOODLE SALAD

NET CARBS
6g

Serves 6

Letting the zoodles sit in a colander with salt before prepping this salad is an important step in the process. If you skip it, your salad might be a little runny.

Calories: 174
Fat: 16g
Sodium: 483mg
Carbohydrates: 8g
Fiber: 2g
Sugar: 4g
Sugar alcohols: 0g
Protein: 3g

INGREDIENTS

3 large zucchini, spiralized

¼ teaspoon sea salt

⅓ cup chopped English cucumber

⅓ cup chopped pitted kalamata olives

⅓ cup chopped cherry tomatoes

2 tablespoons minced red onion

⅓ cup crumbled feta cheese

½ cup Primal Kitchen Greek Vinaigrette & Marinade

1. Place zucchini in a colander over the sink and sprinkle with salt. Let sit for 20 minutes to drain excess water. Pat dry.

2. Transfer zucchini to a large bowl and add cucumber, olives, tomatoes, onion, and feta cheese. Toss to combine.

3. Drizzle vinaigrette on top and toss to coat.

4. Serve immediately.

BACON BROCCOLI SALAD

NET CARBS
7g

Serves 6

Because this broccoli salad doesn't require you to cook the broccoli, you can throw it together in minutes. You can make it up to a week in advance.

Calories: 274
Fat: 20g
Sodium: 516mg
Carbohydrates: 18g
Fiber: 3g
Sugar: 3g
Sugar alcohols: 8g
Protein: 16g

INGREDIENTS

1 large head broccoli, cut into bite-sized florets

½ cup halved cherry tomatoes

8 ounces sharp Cheddar cheese, finely diced

½ cup chopped red onion

8 slices Applegate Naturals No Sugar Bacon, cooked and crumbled

1 cup Tessemae's Organic Mayonnaise

¼ cup Swerve Granular sweetener

2 tablespoons white vinegar

1. Place broccoli in a large bowl.

2. Add tomatoes, cheese, onion, and bacon, and toss to combine.

3. Put mayonnaise, sweetener, and vinegar in a separate small bowl, and whisk to combine. Pour mayonnaise mixture over broccoli mixture and toss to coat evenly.

4. Cover and refrigerate for at least 2 hours before serving.

CAULIFLOWER NO-TATO SALAD

Serves 4

Potato salad is a party and picnic favorite, but traditional versions are loaded with carbohydrates. This keto-friendly version combines all the flavors with the right texture so you won't even realize you're eating cauliflower.

NET CARBS
5g

Calories: 261
Fat: 19g
Sodium: 759mg
Carbohydrates: 8g
Fiber: 3g
Sugar: 3g
Sugar alcohols: 0g
Protein: 16g

INGREDIENTS

4 cups small cauliflower florets

½ cup water

¾ cup Tessemae's Organic Mayonnaise

1 tablespoon yellow mustard

¾ teaspoon celery salt

½ teaspoon ground black pepper

1½ teaspoons dried minced onion

4 large eggs, hard-boiled and chopped

¼ cup chopped Woodstock Organic Kosher Dill Pickles

4 slices Applegate Naturals No Sugar Bacon, cooked and crumbled

¾ cup shredded Cheddar cheese

1. Add cauliflower and water to a large saucepan over medium-high heat. Cover and bring to a boil. Reduce heat to low and steam cauliflower for 8 minutes or until fork-tender. Remove from heat, drain water, and allow to cool for 5 minutes.

2. Combine mayonnaise, mustard, salt, pepper, and dried onion in a large bowl, and whisk until smooth.

3. Add cooked cauliflower, hard-boiled eggs, pickles, bacon, and cheese, and toss to coat evenly.

4. Refrigerate for 2 hours before serving.

CREAMY BROCCOLI AND CAULIFLOWER SOUP

NET CARBS
4g

Calories: 154
Fat: 10g
Sodium: 558mg
Carbohydrates: 6g
Fiber: 2g
Sugar: 2g
Sugar alcohols: 0g
Protein: 11g

Serves 6

If you have an immersion blender, you can use that to blend this soup to your desired consistency instead of transferring it to a regular blender. If you don't have one, consider purchasing one; it's an inexpensive investment that can make life a lot easier when making blended soups.

INGREDIENTS

1 tablespoon salted grass-fed butter

1 medium stalk celery, diced

1 teaspoon minced garlic

4 slices Applegate Naturals No Sugar Bacon, chopped

4 cups Kettle & Fire Classic Chicken Bone Broth

2 cups chopped broccoli

2 cups chopped cauliflower

2 tablespoons no-sugar-added sunflower seed butter

½ teaspoon sea salt

¼ teaspoon cayenne pepper

1 tablespoon dried chives

¼ cup grass-fed heavy cream

1. Heat butter in a large stockpot over medium heat. Add celery and cook until softened, about 4 minutes. Stir in garlic and cook for another 30 seconds.

2. Add bacon and cook until browned and crispy, about 5 minutes.

3. Pour in broth and add broccoli, cauliflower, sunflower seed butter, salt, and cayenne pepper.

4. Reduce heat to low and simmer for 20 minutes. Transfer half the soup to a blender and blend until smooth, about 30 seconds.

5. Pour blended soup back into pot and stir in chives and cream.

6. Remove from heat and allow to cool for 5 minutes, then serve warm.

PORK AND KIMCHI SOUP

Serves 6

You can use any kimchi that you want in this dish, but Wild-brine uses a traditional fermentation method to create high-quality, organic products. Because they're also free of added sugar, most of them are keto-friendly.

INGREDIENTS

2 cups Wildbrine Korean Kimchi

1 tablespoon olive oil

5 cups Kettle & Fire Classic Chicken Bone Broth

1 pound boneless pork shoulder, cut into 1-inch chunks

1 tablespoon Wildbrine Spicy Kimchi Sriracha sauce

¾ teaspoon sea salt

1. Squeeze excess water out of kimchi and set aside on a paper towel.

2. Heat olive oil in a large stockpot over medium heat and add kimchi. Cook for 5 minutes or until kimchi starts to crisp.

3. Add remaining ingredients, stir, and bring to a boil. Reduce heat to low and simmer for 30 minutes or until pork is tender.

4. Remove from heat and serve.

WHAT IS KIMCHI?

Kimchi is a fermented vegetable dish that's similar to sauerkraut. Both fermented dishes are made of cabbage. However, unlike sauerkraut, which generally uses white cabbage and caraway seeds, kimchi is typically made from green cabbage and chili peppers (or chili paste). Like sauerkraut, kimchi is full of beneficial probiotics that keep your gut healthy and can help balance your blood sugar levels.

BUFFALO WING SOUP

Serves 6

If you love buffalo wings, you won't be able to get enough of this soup. It combines creaminess from the cream cheese with just enough heat from the hot sauce to warm you up while satisfying your palate.

NET CARBS
4g

Calories: 277
Fat: 19g
Sodium: 812mg
Carbohydrates: 5g
Fiber: 1g
Sugar: 3g
Sugar alcohols: 0g
Protein: 22g

INGREDIENTS

1 tablespoon salted grass-fed butter

1 small yellow onion, peeled and chopped

1 medium carrot, peeled and diced

1 medium stalk celery, diced

1 teaspoon minced garlic

1 pound boneless, skinless chicken thighs

¼ cup Frank's RedHot Original Cayenne Pepper Sauce

¼ cup Tessemae's Pantry Classic Ranch Dressing & Marinade

4 cups Kettle & Fire Classic Chicken Bone Broth

4 ounces cream cheese, cut into cubes

½ cup crumbled blue cheese

¼ cup chopped green onions

1. Heat butter in a large skillet over medium heat. Add onion, carrot, and celery, and cook until softened, about 4 minutes. Stir in garlic and cook for another 30 seconds.

2. Transfer to a slow cooker and add chicken thighs, pepper sauce, ranch dressing, and broth.

3. Cook on low for 5 hours or until chicken is tender. Remove chicken from slow cooker and shred with two forks. Return to slow cooker, add cream cheese, and stir until cream cheese is melted and smooth. Cook on low for another 30 minutes.

4. Remove from heat and divide among six bowls. Top each serving with equal amounts of blue cheese and green onions.

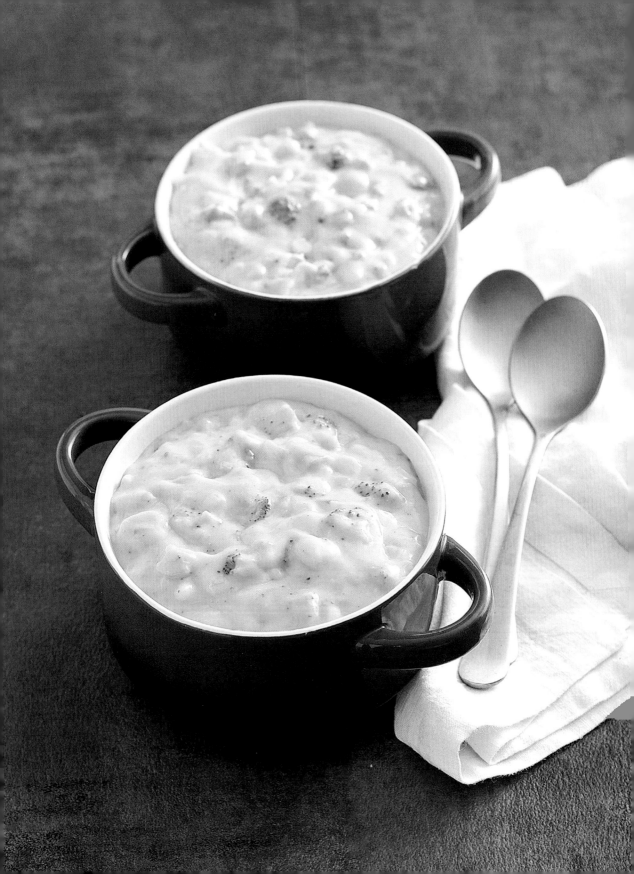

EASY BROCCOLI CHEDDAR SOUP

Serves 6

NET CARBS
8g

Calories: 776
Fat: 70g
Sodium: 751mg
Carbohydrates: 11g
Fiber: 3g
Sugar: 5g
Sugar alcohols: 0g
Protein: 29g

This soup is ready in under 30 minutes and utilizes simple ingredients that you probably already have in your refrigerator and pantry. If you want to save some for later, divide it into freezer-safe containers and freeze it for up to 3 months.

INGREDIENTS

½ cup unsalted grass-fed butter

1 medium yellow onion, peeled and diced

2 teaspoons minced garlic

¾ teaspoon xanthan gum

2 (10-ounce) packages frozen chopped broccoli

4 cups Kettle & Fire Classic Chicken Bone Broth

1 pound shredded Cheddar cheese

2 cups grass-fed heavy cream

½ teaspoon ground black pepper

1. Heat butter in a large stockpot over medium heat. Add onion and cook until softened, about 4 minutes. Add garlic and cook for another minute. Sprinkle xanthan gum over mixture and stir until thickened, about 2 minutes.

2. Stir in broccoli and broth, and reduce heat to low. Simmer until broccoli is bright green and tender, about 10 minutes.

3. Add cheese in ½-cup batches and stir until cheese is melted between each batch. Once cheese is melted and smooth, stir in cream and pepper until incorporated.

4. Remove from heat and serve immediately.

CHICKEN TOMATILLO SOUP

NET CARBS
8g

Serves 6

Once the husks are peeled off, tomatillos look like green tomatoes, but they have a slightly sweet taste, like a cross between a tomato and a strawberry. They're also a more keto-friendly choice than a tomato. One medium tomatillo contains just 1.3 grams of net carbohydrates, while a tomato around the same size contains 3.3 grams of net carbs.

Calories: 247
Fat: 14g
Sodium: 379mg
Carbohydrates: 13g
Fiber: 5g
Sugar: 6g
Sugar alcohols: 0g
Protein: 20g

INGREDIENTS

2 tablespoons olive oil

1 medium yellow onion, peeled and diced

1 teaspoon minced garlic

12 ounces boneless, skinless chicken breasts

1½ pounds tomatillos, peeled and chopped

2 jalapeños, seeded and diced

3 cups Kettle & Fire Classic Chicken Bone Broth

½ teaspoon cayenne pepper

½ teaspoon ground cumin

2 tablespoons chopped fresh parsley

2 teaspoons fresh lime juice

½ teaspoon sea salt

½ teaspoon ground black pepper

¼ cup sour cream

1 medium avocado, peeled, pitted, and thinly sliced

1. Heat olive oil in a medium skillet over medium heat. Add onion and cook until softened, about 4 minutes. Stir in garlic and cook for another 30 seconds. Transfer onion and garlic to a slow cooker.

2. Place chicken in slow cooker and add all remaining ingredients, except sour cream and avocado.

3. Cook on low for 6 hours.

4. Remove chicken from slow cooker and shred with two forks.

5. Transfer vegetables and broth to a blender in batches and blend until smooth. Return to slow cooker.

6. Stir in chicken and cook on low for another 30 minutes.

7. Remove from heat and allow to cool for 5 minutes. Top with sour cream and avocado, then serve warm.

CHEESEBURGER MASON JAR SALAD

Serves 4

Spoiler alert: Thousand Island dressing is often used as a "special sauce" on restaurant burgers. If you want a more basic cheeseburger taste here, you can use no-sugar-added ketchup and mustard in place of the dressing.

Calories: 356
Fat: 26g
Sodium: 1,038mg
Carbohydrates: 6g
Fiber: 1g
Sugar: 2g
Sugar alcohols: 0g
Protein: 23g

INGREDIENTS

1 pound 85/15 ground beef

1 teaspoon sea salt

¼ teaspoon ground black pepper

½ teaspoon garlic powder

½ teaspoon onion powder

½ cup Primal Kitchen Thousand Island Dressing & Marinade

¼ cup minced yellow onion

¼ cup diced tomatoes

¼ cup minced Woodstock Organic Kosher Dill Pickles

¼ cup shredded Cheddar cheese

4 cups chopped romaine lettuce

1. Heat a large skillet over medium-high heat. Crumble beef into skillet and add salt, pepper, garlic powder, and onion powder. Cook until beef is no longer pink, about 8 minutes. Remove from heat and allow to cool to room temperature.

2. Pour 2 tablespoons dressing in the bottom of each of four widemouthed quart-sized Mason jars.

3. In each jar, layer one-fourth of the beef, 1 tablespoon onion, 1 tablespoon tomatoes, 1 tablespoon pickles, 1 tablespoon cheese, and 1 cup chopped lettuce.

4. Cover and store in the refrigerator until ready to eat, up to 1 week.

5. When ready to eat, shake vigorously to combine ingredients and coat with dressing.

LAYERING YOUR MASON JAR SALAD

When layering a Mason jar salad, always put the dressing on the bottom, then layer the rest of it according to weight. The heaviest ingredients, like meat or chicken, go in first, followed by the medium-weight ingredients, like tomatoes or pickles, and then the lettuce or whatever greens you're using. This keeps everything nicely separated so that the greens stay crisp until you're ready to eat them.

KALE AND SALMON SALAD

Serves 2

Baby kale isn't as tough as regular kale, and it has a milder taste too. Because of that, it's a great choice for salads and any other dish that calls for raw kale. If you're not a fan of kale in any form, you can use baby spinach in its place.

Calories: 806
Fat: 74g
Sodium: 669mg
Carbohydrates: 13g
Fiber: 8g
Sugar: 2g
Sugar alcohols: 0g
Protein: 27g

INGREDIENTS

6 tablespoons olive oil, divided

1 teaspoon minced garlic

1 (8-ounce) wild Alaskan salmon fillet, skin removed

½ teaspoon sea salt

¼ teaspoon ground black pepper

1 tablespoon fresh lemon juice

4 cups chopped baby kale

1 large avocado, peeled, pitted, and diced

1 tablespoon pine nuts

2 tablespoons apple cider vinegar

1. Heat 2 tablespoons olive oil in a large skillet over medium heat. Add garlic and sauté for 3 minutes.

2. Season salmon with salt and pepper and add to skillet. Cook for 4 minutes on each side or until fish flakes easily with a fork. Drizzle lemon juice on top. Remove from heat and cut in half.

3. Divide kale between two plates and top each plate with half of the avocado, ½ tablespoon pine nuts, and half the salmon.

4. In a separate small bowl, combine remaining olive oil and apple cider vinegar. Pour half of mixture over each plate. Serve immediately.

LOBSTER BISQUE

Serves 6

This Lobster Bisque is best with freshly cooked lobster meat, but if you don't have the extra time or fresh lobster available near you, you can find frozen lobster meat in many grocery store freezers. A high-quality, wild-caught lobster meat is best.

INGREDIENTS

⅓ cup unsalted grass-fed butter

1 large yellow onion, peeled and diced

½ teaspoon xanthan gum

¾ teaspoon celery salt

¼ teaspoon ground black pepper

2 cups Kettle & Fire Classic Chicken Bone Broth

4 cups grass-fed heavy cream

3 cups cooked lobster meat

1. Heat butter in a large stockpot over medium heat. Add onion and cook for 5 minutes. Add xanthan gum, celery salt, and pepper, and stir until thickened, about 2 minutes.

2. Reduce heat to low and stir in broth and cream. Cook until thickened, about 5 minutes, whisking frequently.

3. Add lobster and cook for an additional 10 minutes.

4. Remove from heat and allow to cool for 5 minutes, then serve warm.

HEALTH BENEFITS OF LOBSTER

Lobster has some pretty amazing health benefits. In addition to being high in omega-3 fatty acids, lobster is a rich source of iodine, a mineral that helps keep your thyroid gland functioning properly. A single 3.5-ounce serving of lobster contains about 71 percent of the total iodine that you need for the whole day.

SALMON COBB MASON JAR SALAD

Serves 4

The salmon adds a significant amount of omega-3 fatty acids to this salad. You can cook some fresh fillets instead of using canned salmon if you prefer, or use another protein source instead; but keep in mind that doing so will change the nutritional content.

NET CARBS
5g

Calories: 417
Fat: 31g
Sodium: 1,010mg
Carbohydrates: 7g
Fiber: 2g
Sugar: 4g
Sugar alcohols: 0g
Protein: 28g

INGREDIENTS

½ cup Tessemae's Organic Creamy Ranch Dressing

2 (6-ounce) cans wild Alaskan pink salmon, drained

½ cup chopped hard-boiled egg

½ cup chopped cooked Applegate Naturals No Sugar Bacon

½ cup chopped avocado

½ cup crumbled blue cheese

½ cup chopped grape tomatoes

¼ cup minced red onion

4 cups chopped iceberg lettuce

1. Put 2 tablespoons dressing in the bottom of each of four quart-sized widemouthed Mason jars.

2. Layer 3 ounces salmon, 2 tablespoons hard-boiled egg, 2 tablespoons bacon, 2 tablespoons avocado, 2 tablespoons blue cheese, 2 tablespoons tomatoes, 1 tablespoon red onion, and 1 cup lettuce in each jar.

3. Cover and refrigerate until ready to eat, up to 1 week.

4. When ready to eat, shake vigorously to combine ingredients and coat with dressing.

GETTING YOUR OMEGA-3S

Omega-3 fatty acids are classified as essential fats because, unlike other fats, your body can't make them; you have to get them from your diet. They're highly important because they affect the function of all your cells. Omega-3 fats play huge roles in preventing heart disease and stroke and reducing inflammation. Salmon is one of the richest sources, offering a whopping 2,260 milligrams per 3.5 ounces. Most health experts recommend getting between 250 and 500 milligrams per day.

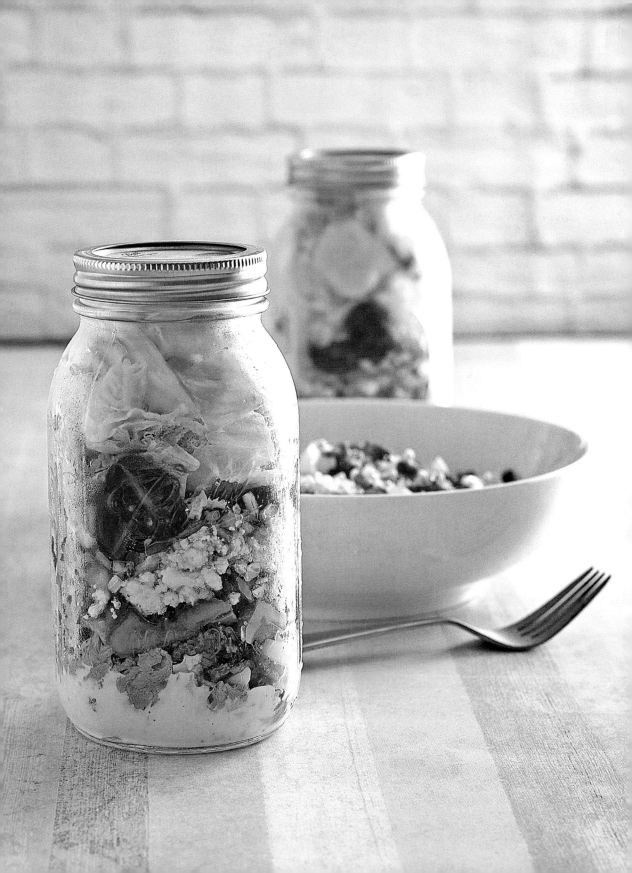

BACON TURKEY CLUB MASON JAR SALAD

Serves 6

Always make sure to check your deli meat labels! Sugar and other sweeteners are often hidden in deli meats to make them last longer. If you're getting them from the deli counter, ask if you can read the ingredient list before ordering to make sure the meat fits into your keto diet plan.

INGREDIENTS

¾ cup Tessemae's Organic Habanero Ranch Dressing

1½ cups cherry tomatoes, halved

12 slices Applegate Naturals No Sugar Bacon, cooked and crumbled

1½ pounds sliced Applegate Organics Oven Roasted Turkey Breast, chopped

¾ cup shredded Cheddar cheese

6 cups chopped romaine lettuce

1. Pour 2 tablespoons dressing in the bottom of each of six quart-sized widemouthed Mason jars.

2. Layer ¼ cup tomatoes, one-sixth of the crumbled bacon, 4 ounces chopped turkey, 2 tablespoons cheese, and 1 cup lettuce in each jar.

3. Cover and refrigerate until ready to eat, up to 1 week.

4. When ready to eat, shake vigorously to combine ingredients and coat with dressing.

JALAPEÑO CHEDDAR SOUP

Serves 6

Make sure you use fresh jalapeño peppers for this recipe, not the pickled jalapeños that come in a jar. And don't forget to use gloves when chopping them! That will protect your skin from the spice and ensure that you don't get any in your eyes later if you rub them.

NET CARBS
5g

Calories: 761
Fat: 60g
Sodium: 1,328mg
Carbohydrates: 6g
Fiber: 1g
Sugar: 3g
Sugar alcohols: 0g
Protein: 81g

INGREDIENTS

2 tablespoons salted grass-fed butter

1 medium yellow onion, peeled and finely diced

1 cup chopped celery

1 cup diced fresh jalapeño

1 teaspoon minced garlic

1 teaspoon xanthan gum

5 cups Kettle & Fire Classic Chicken Bone Broth

2 pounds shredded sharp Cheddar cheese

3 tablespoons grass-fed heavy cream

½ teaspoon ground white pepper

1. Heat butter in a large stockpot over medium heat. Add onion and celery and cook until softened, about 4 minutes. Add jalapeño and cook for another 3 minutes. Stir in garlic and cook until fragrant, about 30 seconds.

2. Stir in xanthan gum and cook for an additional minute.

3. Slowly pour in broth, whisking mixture as you go. Reduce heat to low and simmer for 15 minutes to allow mixture to thicken.

4. Add cheese a little bit at a time, stirring to incorporate each batch before you add more. When cheese is melted and smooth, stir in cream and white pepper.

5. Remove from heat and serve immediately.

CHAPTER 5

POULTRY

PARMESAN-CRUSTED CHICKEN TENDERS

Serves 6

If you don't have boneless chicken tenders, you can use boneless, skinless chicken breasts and slice them into thinner pieces. You can also turn this into an appetizer by using bite-sized pieces of chicken and following the rest of the recipe as written.

Calories: 262
Fat: 12g
Sodium: 385mg
Carbohydrates: 1g
Fiber: 0g
Sugar: 0g
Sugar alcohols: 0g
Protein: 36g

INGREDIENTS

¾ cup crushed EPIC Oven Baked Pink Himalayan and Sea Salt Pork Rinds

¼ cup grated Parmesan cheese

1 teaspoon garlic powder

1 teaspoon onion powder

½ teaspoon dried parsley

¼ teaspoon crushed red pepper flakes

¼ teaspoon sea salt

¼ teaspoon ground black pepper

2 large eggs

1½ pounds boneless, skinless chicken tenders

2 tablespoons Nutiva Organic Coconut Oil with Buttery Flavor

1. Combine pork rinds, cheese, garlic powder, onion powder, parsley, red pepper flakes, salt, and black pepper in a shallow dish. Set aside.

2. Add eggs to a small bowl and whisk lightly.

3. Dip each chicken tender into eggs and then press into pork rind mixture, coating both sides evenly.

4. Heat coconut oil in a large skillet over medium-high heat. Add coated chicken tenders to skillet and cook for 4 minutes on each side or until chicken is no longer pink.

5. Transfer to a paper towel–lined plate to absorb excess oil.

6. Serve warm.

BUFFALO BLUE CHEESE CHICKEN BURGERS

Serves 6

If you're not a fan of the distinct flavor of blue cheese, you can swap it for feta cheese with equally delicious results. Serve with your favorite burger toppings (minus the bun) and some keto-friendly ranch dressing to dip.

Calories: 375
Fat: 27g
Sodium: 771mg
Carbohydrates: 6g
Fiber: 3g
Sugar: 2g
Sugar alcohols: 0g
Protein: 30g

INGREDIENTS

1½ pounds ground chicken

1½ cups coarse almond meal

¾ cup crumbled blue cheese

1 large egg, lightly beaten

2 tablespoons dried minced onion

½ cup Frank's RedHot Original Cayenne Pepper Sauce

1. Combine all ingredients in a large bowl and mix with your hands until incorporated. Refrigerate for 1 hour.

2. Preheat oven to 350°F. Line a baking sheet with parchment paper and set aside.

3. Form chicken mixture into six patties and transfer to prepared baking sheet.

4. Bake for 20 minutes or until chicken reaches an internal temperature of 165°F, flipping once during cooking.

5. Remove from oven. Allow to cool for 5 minutes, then serve warm.

GROUND TURKEY AND ZUCCHINI RICE BOWL

NET CARBS

6g

Serves 6

This recipe is perfect for a quick weeknight meal and is easy to make ahead of time. You can change it up a little bit by using different vegetables, like broccoli or spinach, and different ground meats (chicken, beef, and pork also work well).

Calories: 324
Fat: 12g
Sodium: 629mg
Carbohydrates: 8g
Fiber: 2g
Sugar: 3g
Sugar alcohols: 0g
Protein: 21g

INGREDIENTS

1 tablespoon olive oil

1 teaspoon minced garlic

1 medium yellow onion, peeled and diced

1½ pounds ground turkey

1 large zucchini, sliced into coins and quartered

1 (10-ounce) package frozen cauliflower rice

1 teaspoon garlic powder

1 teaspoon onion powder

1 teaspoon sea salt

1 teaspoon ground black pepper

½ teaspoon paprika

1 teaspoon dried parsley

¼ cup plus 2 tablespoons Tessemae's Organic Habanero Ranch Dressing

1. Heat olive oil in a medium skillet over medium heat.

2. Add garlic and cook for 1 minute. Add onion and cook for an additional 4 minutes or until onion is softened. Crumble in turkey and cook until no longer pink, about 7 minutes.

3. Stir in zucchini and cauliflower rice. Sprinkle garlic powder, onion powder, salt, pepper, paprika, and parsley on top, and stir to combine. Cover and cook until cauliflower rice is softened, about 5 minutes.

4. Remove from heat and transfer to bowls.

5. Top each serving with 1 tablespoon dressing and serve.

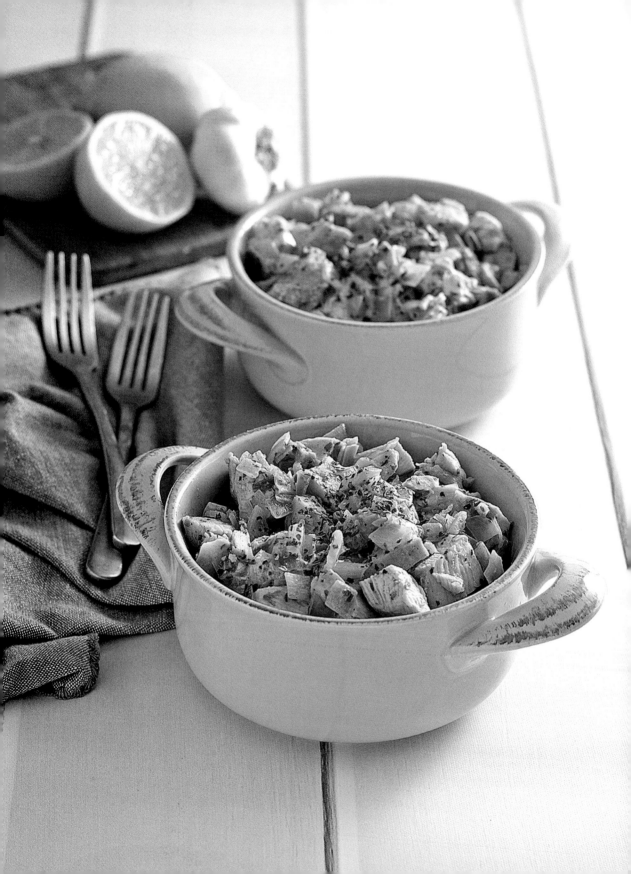

LEMON GARLIC CHICKEN

Serves 6

This Lemon Garlic Chicken doesn't require any fancy ingredients, but it tastes like it came from a fancy restaurant. If you don't have arrowroot powder, you can use ¼ teaspoon of xanthan gum in its place.

Calories: 223
Fat: 11g
Sodium: 365mg
Carbohydrates: 4g
Fiber: 1g
Sugar: 1g
Sugar alcohols: 0g
Protein: 26g

INGREDIENTS

½ teaspoon sea salt

½ teaspoon ground black pepper

¼ teaspoon paprika

1 teaspoon garlic powder

¼ teaspoon onion salt

1½ pounds boneless, skinless chicken breasts, cubed

1 tablespoon olive oil

2 tablespoons salted grass-fed butter

1 small yellow onion, peeled and roughly chopped

1½ teaspoons minced garlic

¼ cup Kettle & Fire Classic Chicken Bone Broth

1 teaspoon dried oregano

1 teaspoon dried basil

2 tablespoons fresh lemon juice

1 teaspoon lemon zest

2 tablespoons Native Forest Organic Heavy Coconut Cream

2 tablespoons water

2 teaspoons arrowroot powder

1. Combine salt, pepper, paprika, garlic powder, and onion salt in a large bowl. Add chicken to bowl and toss to coat.

2. Turn pressure cooker to sauté function and heat olive oil. Add chicken and cook until browned, about 5 minutes. Remove chicken from pot and set aside.

3. Add butter, chopped onion, and minced garlic to pot, and cook for 2 minutes, stirring and scraping the bottom of the pot to remove browned bits from the bottom. Add broth, oregano, basil, lemon juice, and lemon zest, and stir to combine.

4. Return chicken to pot and secure lid. Cook on high pressure for 7 minutes. Allow pressure to release naturally for 3 minutes and then release any remaining pressure manually. Remove lid.

5. Allow to cool for 5 minutes, then stir in coconut cream. Combine water and arrowroot powder in a small bowl, then stir into sauce.

6. Cool for another 3 minutes. Serve hot.

WHAT'S NATURAL PRESSURE RELEASE?

When a pressure cooker recipe calls for natural release, it means that you should let the pressure release on its own, rather than turning the valve to release the pressure. Allowing the pressure to release naturally typically lets the food cook longer.

GARLIC AND HERB–ROASTED TURKEY

Serves 8

Cooking a whole turkey isn't something that needs to be exclusive to Thanksgiving. Roasting a whole bird is actually an easy way to feed a crowd *and* save leftovers for some easy keto meals for the rest of your week.

NET CARBS
4g

Calories: 808
Fat: 43g
Sodium: 727mg
Carbohydrates: 4g
Fiber: 0g
Sugar: 0g
Sugar alcohols: 0g
Protein: 96g

INGREDIENTS

½ cup salted grass-fed butter, softened

½ teaspoon dried thyme

4 teaspoons minced garlic

2 heads garlic, cut in half crosswise

6 sprigs fresh thyme

2 slices fresh lemon

¼ cup olive oil

1 (12-pound) whole turkey

1 teaspoon sea salt

1 teaspoon cracked black pepper

1. Preheat oven to 425°F.

2. Combine butter, dried thyme, and minced garlic in a small bowl, and stir until smooth. Set aside.

3. Arrange the cut garlic heads on the bottom of a large roasting pan (cut side down). Add fresh thyme and lemon slices and pour in olive oil.

4. Rub butter mixture all over turkey, including underneath the skin, then season with salt and pepper. Transfer turkey to roasting pan.

5. Roast uncovered for 30 minutes. Reduce heat to 325°F and continue roasting for 2 hours or until internal temperature reaches 165°F.

6. Remove from oven and tent with foil. Allow to rest for 30 minutes, then carve and serve.

CHICKEN FAJITA SKILLET

Serves 6

NET CARBS
6g

Instead of pairing these chicken fajitas with flour tortillas, which are full of processed carbs, serve them with a side of cauliflower rice, made Mexican-style with chopped green chiles, tomato paste, cumin, and paprika. You'll still get that starchy feel (and fullness), but with considerably fewer carbs.

Calories: 221
Fat: 8g
Sodium: 423mg
Carbohydrates: 9g
Fiber: 3g
Sugar: 4g
Sugar alcohols: 0g
Protein: 27g

INGREDIENTS

2 tablespoons olive oil

1 cup chopped green bell pepper

1 cup chopped red bell pepper

1 cup diced onion

1½ pounds thinly sliced boneless, skinless chicken tenders

1½ teaspoons chili powder

1 teaspoon ground cumin

½ teaspoon paprika

½ teaspoon sea salt

¼ teaspoon ground black pepper

1 (14.5-ounce) can petite-diced tomatoes, drained

1 (4.5-ounce) can diced green chiles

1. Heat olive oil in a large skillet over medium heat. Add peppers and onion, and cook until softened, about 5 minutes. Remove from skillet and set aside.

2. Add chicken to skillet. Sprinkle with chili powder, cumin, paprika, salt, and black pepper. Cook until chicken is no longer pink, about 6 minutes.

3. Return onion and peppers to skillet and add tomatoes and green chiles. Cook for another 2 minutes.

4. Remove from heat and serve immediately.

CHEESE-STUFFED CHICKEN MEATBALLS

NET CARBS
1g

Calories: 311
Fat: 22g
Sodium: 622mg
Carbohydrates: 2g
Fiber: 1g
Sugar: 1g
Sugar alcohols: 0g
Protein: 27g

Serves 5

The pepper jack cheese in this recipe gives these meatballs a little kick, but if you prefer a milder taste, you can swap it out for cubes of Cheddar, mozzarella, or Monterey jack cheese with equally delicious results.

INGREDIENTS

1 pound ground chicken

⅓ cup almond flour

¾ teaspoon sea salt

1 teaspoon garlic powder

½ teaspoon onion powder

½ teaspoon dried parsley

1 large egg, lightly beaten

6 ounces pepper jack cheese, cubed into 20 pieces

1. Preheat oven to 400°F. Line a baking sheet with parchment paper and set aside.

2. Combine all ingredients, except for cheese, in a large bowl.

3. Form a small portion of the mixture into a 1½-inch ball around a cube of cheese. Place on prepared baking sheet.

4. Repeat with remaining mixture. You should end up with twenty meatballs.

5. Transfer to oven and bake for 25 minutes or until cooked through.

6. Remove from oven and allow to cool for 5 minutes, then serve warm.

ASIAN-INSPIRED TURKEY RICE BOWL

NET CARBS
4g

Serves 6

This recipe combines traditional Asian flavors like soy, sesame, and ginger in a keto-friendly bowl that uses coconut aminos in place of the soy sauce.

Calories: 206
Fat: 14g
Sodium: 262mg
Carbohydrates: 14g
Fiber: 2g
Sugar: 3g
Sugar alcohols: 8g
Protein: 14g

INGREDIENTS

¼ cup Swerve Brown sweetener

¼ cup coconut aminos

2 teaspoons sesame oil

½ teaspoon crushed red pepper flakes

¼ teaspoon ground ginger

1 tablespoon coconut oil

2 teaspoons minced garlic

1 small yellow onion, peeled and finely chopped

1 pound ground turkey

2 large green onions, trimmed and chopped

1 teaspoon sesame seeds

1 (10-ounce) package frozen cauliflower rice, cooked to manufacturer's instructions

1. Combine sweetener, coconut aminos, sesame oil, red pepper flakes, and ginger in a small bowl, and whisk until sweetener is incorporated. Set aside.

2. Heat coconut oil in a large skillet over medium heat. Add garlic and yellow onion, and cook for 3 minutes. Crumble turkey into skillet and cook until no longer pink, about 7 minutes.

3. Stir in coconut aminos mixture and cook for another minute. Add green onions and sesame seeds and cook for another minute.

4. Remove from heat and serve over prepared cauliflower rice.

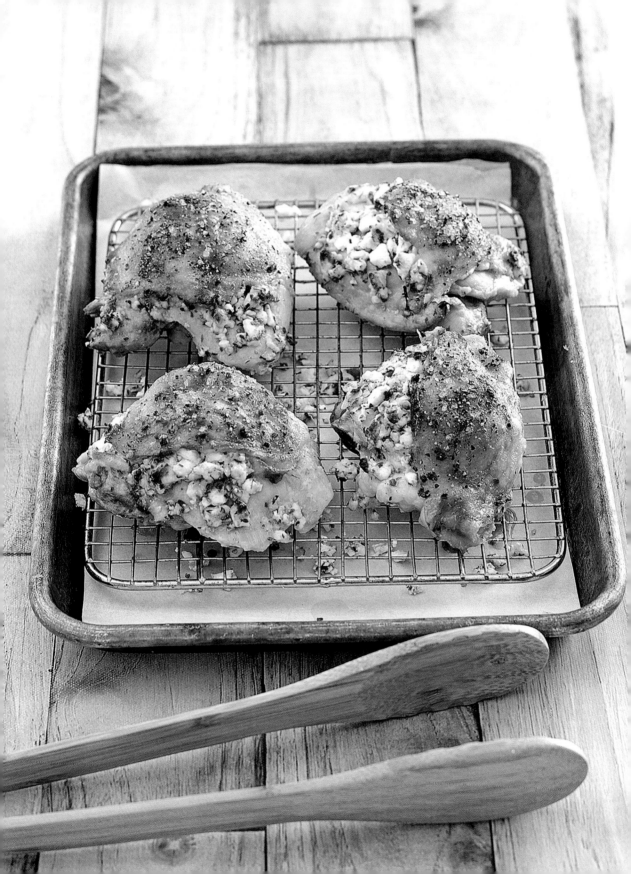

GARLIC FETA–BAKED CHICKEN THIGHS

Serves 6

Chicken thighs are a little higher in fat than chicken breasts (and a little more flavorful because of that), but if you prefer white meat, you can simply swap the thighs for breasts and follow the rest of the recipe as written.

INGREDIENTS

4 ounces crumbled feta cheese

2 teaspoons minced garlic

¼ teaspoon crushed red pepper flakes

2 teaspoons ground black pepper, divided

2 teaspoons dried oregano

2 teaspoons olive oil

1½ pounds bone-in, skin-on chicken thighs

1 tablespoon unsalted grass-fed butter, melted

1 teaspoon sea salt

1. Preheat oven to 400°F. Line a baking sheet with parchment paper and set aside.

2. Combine feta cheese, garlic, red pepper flakes, 1 teaspoon black pepper, oregano, and olive oil in a small bowl and mix until smooth.

3. Pull skin away from chicken thighs and spread feta cheese mixture evenly under the skin.

4. Arrange chicken thighs on prepared baking sheet and drizzle melted butter on top. Sprinkle salt and remaining 1 teaspoon black pepper on each thigh.

5. Bake for 35 minutes or until juices run clear.

6. Remove from oven and allow to cool for 5 minutes, then serve warm.

PARMESAN AND HERB–CRUSTED TURKEY TENDERLOIN

NET CARBS
0g

Calories: 130
Fat: 2g
Sodium: 471mg
Carbohydrates: 0g
Fiber: 0g
Sugar: 0g
Sugar alcohols: 0g
Protein: 28g

Serves 6

If you can't find turkey tenderloin in your grocery store, you can either make a special request with your local butcher or swap it out for pork tenderloin instead. Pork is a bit higher in fat and has a mild flavor that also works well with this combo of herbs and spices.

INGREDIENTS

1½ pounds boneless, skinless turkey tenderloin

2 tablespoons Tessemae's Organic Mayonnaise

1 tablespoon shredded Parmesan cheese

1 tablespoon lemon zest

1 teaspoon minced garlic

1 teaspoon dried rosemary

1 teaspoon dried oregano

1 teaspoon dried parsley

1 teaspoon sea salt

½ teaspoon ground black pepper

1. Preheat oven to 400°F. Spray a 9" × 13" baking pan with cooking spray.

2. Arrange turkey tenderloin in prepared baking pan.

3. Combine mayonnaise, cheese, lemon zest, garlic, rosemary, oregano, and parsley in a small bowl and mix until smooth.

4. Spread mayonnaise mixture evenly over tenderloin. Sprinkle with salt and pepper.

5. Bake for 35 minutes or until internal temperature reaches 160°F.

6. Remove from oven and allow to rest for 10 minutes, then slice and serve warm.

TURKEY BACON CHEESE-BURGER MEATLOAF

Serves 6

The bacon and cheese in this meatloaf keep the ground turkey nice and moist. Make sure to watch the meatloaf closely so that it doesn't overcook, though. The best way to monitor temperature is with a meat thermometer. Ground turkey is done when the internal temperature hits 165°F.

Calories: 295
Fat: 21g
Sodium: 1,380mg
Carbohydrates: 4g
Fiber: 0g
Sugar: 2g
Sugar alcohols: 0g
Protein: 22g

INGREDIENTS

- 1 (8-ounce) package Applegate Naturals No Sugar Bacon, cooked and crumbled
- 1 pound ground turkey
- 1 cup shredded Cheddar cheese
- 1 large egg, lightly beaten
- ½ small yellow onion, peeled and diced
- 1 tablespoon coconut aminos
- 2 teaspoons garlic powder
- ½ teaspoon sea salt
- ¼ teaspoon ground black pepper
- ¼ cup Tessemae's Unsweetened Ketchup
- 2 tablespoons yellow mustard

1. Preheat oven to 350°F. Line an 8" × 4" loaf pan with parchment paper and set aside.

2. Combine all ingredients except ketchup and mustard in a large bowl, and mix with your hands until fully incorporated.

3. Transfer mixture to prepared loaf pan.

4. Whisk ketchup and mustard together in a small bowl until smooth. Spread evenly on top of meatloaf.

5. Bake for 55 minutes or until internal temperature reaches 165°F.

6. Remove from oven and allow to cool for 5 minutes, then slice and serve.

CURRIED GROUND TURKEY

Serves 4

This easy weeknight meal combines all the flavors of a rich curry in a simple, one-pan recipe. If you want to raise the fat content a bit, you can use a mixture of ground turkey and ground beef. Serve over cauliflower rice or with a side of roasted broccoli.

NET CARBS
4g

Calories: 318
Fat: 23g
Sodium: 757mg
Carbohydrates: 7g
Fiber: 3g
Sugar: 3g
Sugar alcohols: 0g
Protein: 21g

INGREDIENTS

2 teaspoons coconut oil

1 small yellow onion, peeled and minced

1½ teaspoons minced garlic

1 pound ground turkey

1½ tablespoons curry powder

1½ teaspoons ground cumin

1½ teaspoons ground coriander

1 teaspoon ground turmeric

½ teaspoon ground ginger

1 teaspoon sea salt

1 tablespoon tomato paste

1 (14.5-ounce) can petite-diced tomatoes

½ cup full-fat coconut milk

1. Heat coconut oil in a large skillet over medium heat.

2. Add onion and cook for 5 minutes or until softened. Add garlic and cook for another minute or until fragrant.

3. Crumble ground turkey into skillet and cook until no longer pink, about 7 minutes.

4. Combine curry powder, cumin, coriander, turmeric, ginger, and salt in a small bowl. Sprinkle over turkey mixture and stir to incorporate.

5. Add remaining ingredients and stir until smooth.

6. Turn heat to low and simmer for 3 minutes or until sauce thickens slightly.

7. Remove from heat and serve immediately.

CREAM CHEESE–STUFFED CHICKEN CUTLETS

NET CARBS
3g

Calories: 266
Fat: 15g
Sodium: 553mg
Carbohydrates: 4g
Fiber: 1g
Sugar: 2g
Sugar alcohols: 0g
Protein: 29g

Serves 6

Cream cheese makes a nice, thick filling that's perfect for chicken, but if you don't have any on hand, you can use a keto-friendly mayonnaise in its place. If you do use mayonnaise, you'll save yourself a small amount of carbs too.

INGREDIENTS

1 tablespoon salted grass-fed butter

8 ounces white mushrooms, roughly chopped

2 cups chopped fresh spinach

2 teaspoons minced garlic

6 ounces cream cheese, softened

1½ pounds boneless, skinless chicken cutlets

1 teaspoon sea salt

½ teaspoon ground black pepper

½ teaspoon garlic powder

1. Preheat oven to 400°F. Line a baking sheet with parchment paper and set aside.

2. Heat butter in a large skillet over medium heat. Add mushrooms and cook until softened, about 5 minutes. Add spinach and cook for another 2 minutes or until spinach is wilted. Stir minced garlic and cream cheese into skillet, and cook until cream cheese is melted and everything is combined, about 3 minutes.

3. Remove from heat and set aside.

4. Pound chicken cutlets with a meat mallet until ⅛" thick. Spread equal amounts cream cheese mixture onto each chicken cutlet, then roll them up and secure with a toothpick in each.

5. Transfer rolled cutlets to prepared baking sheet and sprinkle with salt, pepper, and garlic powder.

6. Bake for 15 minutes or until juices run clear.

7. Remove from oven and serve immediately.

FOUR-CHEESE WHITE PIZZA

NET CARBS
6g

Serves 6

This Four-Cheese White Pizza uses a low-carb, fat-rich Alfredo sauce in place of the tomato sauce of traditional pizza. You can play around with adding other low-carb toppings too!

Calories: 541
Fat: 44g
Sodium: 649mg
Carbohydrates: 10g
Fiber: 4g
Sugar: 3g
Sugar alcohols: 0g
Protein: 29g

INGREDIENTS

For the pizza crust:

1½ cups whole milk mozzarella cheese

2 ounces cream cheese

1 large egg, lightly beaten

1½ cups almond flour

½ teaspoon garlic powder

For the sauce:

2 tablespoons salted grass-fed butter

1 teaspoon minced garlic

½ cup grass-fed heavy cream

1 ounce cream cheese, softened

⅛ teaspoon sea salt

⅛ teaspoon ground white pepper

1/16 teaspoon ground nutmeg

⅓ cup grated Parmesan cheese

1. To make the pizza crust, preheat oven to 400°F.

2. Combine mozzarella cheese and cream cheese in a microwave-safe bowl. Microwave on high for 60 seconds, stir, and then microwave for another 60 seconds or until cheese is melted. Stir well.

3. Transfer cheeses to a food processor and add remaining crust ingredients. Pulse until a dough forms.

4. Transfer dough to a piece of parchment paper and cover with another piece of parchment paper. Use a rolling pin to roll dough out into a 12" × 15" rectangle and remove the top piece of parchment paper.

5. Pick the dough up with the bottom piece of parchment paper and transfer to a baking sheet.

6. Use a fork to poke holes in the dough and bake for 9 minutes or until lightly golden.

7. While crust is baking, make the sauce: Melt butter in a large skillet over medium heat. Add garlic and cook for 1 minute. Add heavy cream, cream cheese, salt, pepper, and nutmeg, and reduce heat to low.

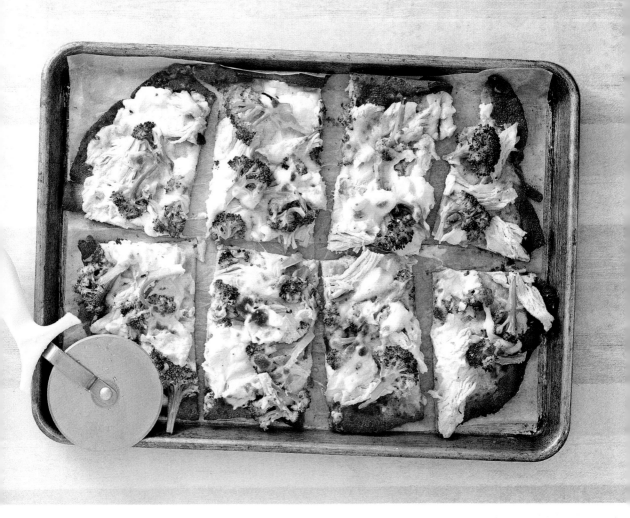

For the toppings:

½ cup whole milk ricotta cheese

¾ cup cooked chopped broccoli

1 cup cooked diced boneless, skinless chicken breasts

1 cup shredded whole milk mozzarella cheese

8. Continue cooking until cream cheese melts and sauce is smooth. Slowly whisk in Parmesan cheese, stirring until sauce thickens, about 5 minutes. Remove from heat.

9. When dough is done baking, remove from oven and spread sauce evenly on top. Dollop ricotta cheese on top of sauce and evenly spread broccoli and chicken on top of pizza. Sprinkle mozzarella cheese over entire pizza.

10. Bake for 12 minutes or until cheese is bubbly and starting to brown. Remove from oven and allow to cool for 5 minutes, then serve warm.

CHICKEN, BACON, AND RANCH CASSEROLE

Serves 6

This recipe freezes and reheats really well, so don't be afraid to double up on your ingredients when making it. You can make two casseroles and save one for a night when you want to get a keto-friendly dinner on the table without any hands-on work. To reheat, cook the frozen casserole at 375°F for 75 minutes.

INGREDIENTS

- 1½ pounds boneless, skinless chicken thighs, cooked and cubed
- 6 slices Applegate Naturals No Sugar Bacon, cooked and crumbled
- 1½ cups frozen broccoli, thawed
- 1 teaspoon minced garlic
- ½ cup Tessemae's Pantry Classic Ranch Dressing & Marinade
- ¼ cup shredded Parmesan cheese
- 1 cup shredded whole milk mozzarella cheese, divided
- 1 cup shredded Cheddar cheese, divided

1. Preheat oven to 375°F.

2. Place chicken, bacon, broccoli, garlic, dressing, Parmesan cheese, ½ cup mozzarella cheese, and ½ cup Cheddar cheese in a large bowl. Stir to coat chicken evenly.

3. Transfer chicken mixture to an ungreased 9" × 13" dish, and sprinkle remaining mozzarella and Cheddar cheese on top.

4. Bake for 20 minutes or until cheese is melted and casserole is hot and bubbly.

5. Remove from oven and allow to cool for 5 minutes, then serve warm.

ZESTY BARBECUE CHICKEN

Serves 6

If you're not using Primal Kitchen products, make sure that both the barbecue sauce and the Italian dressing that you use for this recipe don't have any added sugar. Most store-bought barbecue sauces are loaded with sweeteners that aren't keto-friendly.

INGREDIENTS

- 1½ pounds boneless, skinless chicken breasts
- ½ cup diced yellow onion
- 2 cups Primal Kitchen Classic BBQ Sauce, Organic and Unsweetened
- ½ cup Primal Kitchen Italian Vinaigrette & Marinade
- 2 tablespoons coconut aminos

1. Place chicken and onion in a slow cooker. Combine remaining ingredients in a medium bowl and pour over chicken and onion.

2. Cover and cook on low for 7 hours or until chicken is cooked through (use a meat thermometer to check for doneness) and tender.

3. Remove chicken from slow cooker, shred with two forks, and return to slow cooker. Stir and allow to cook for another hour.

4. Allow to cool for 5 minutes, then serve warm.

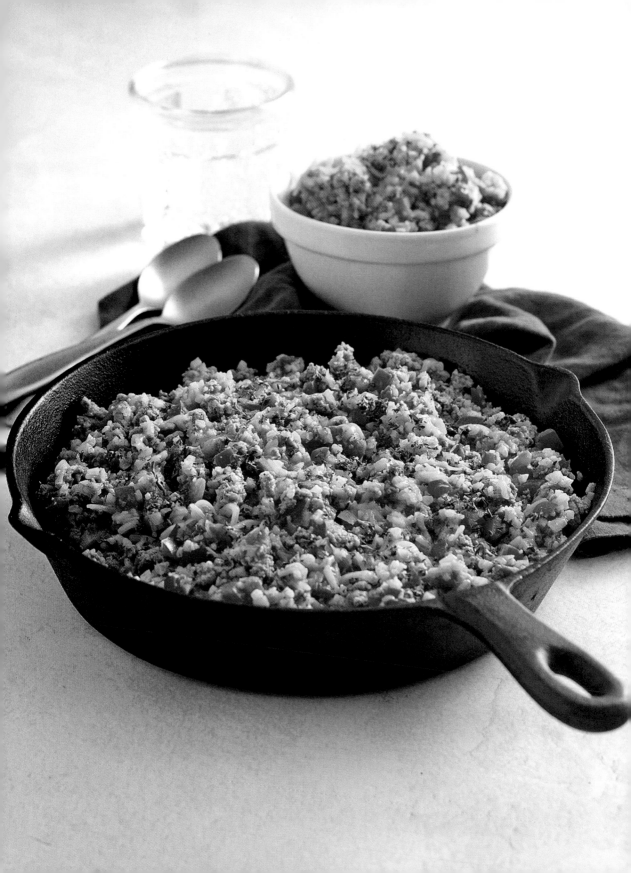

DECONSTRUCTED STUFFED PEPPER BOWLS

NET CARBS
7g

Calories: 318
Fat: 21g
Sodium: 724mg
Carbohydrates: 12g
Fiber: 5g
Sugar: 5g
Sugar alcohols: 0g
Protein: 20g

Serves 6

This recipe combines all the flavors of stuffed peppers but eliminates the hassle of blanching the peppers after baking. You can use green peppers, yellow peppers, or orange peppers in place of the red ones with only a negligible change in the carb count.

INGREDIENTS

- 2 tablespoons olive oil
- 1 small yellow onion, peeled and diced
- 2 cups chopped red bell peppers
- 1 teaspoon minced garlic
- 1 pound ground turkey
- 1 teaspoon sea salt
- ½ teaspoon ground black pepper
- 1½ teaspoons chili powder
- 1½ teaspoons ground cumin
- ½ teaspoon paprika
- 1 teaspoon dried parsley
- 1 tablespoon tomato paste
- 1 (14.5-ounce) can fire-roasted diced tomatoes
- 2 (10-ounce) packages frozen cauliflower rice
- 1 cup shredded Cheddar cheese

1. Heat olive oil in a large skillet over medium heat. Add onion and bell peppers, and cook until softened, about 5 minutes. Add garlic and cook for 1 more minute.

2. Crumble turkey into skillet and cook for 2 minutes. Sprinkle with salt, black pepper, chili powder, cumin, paprika, and parsley. Cook until turkey is no longer pink, about 5 more minutes.

3. Stir in tomato paste and diced tomatoes. Add cauliflower rice and stir to combine. Cover and cook until softened, about 7 minutes.

4. Sprinkle cheese on top and stir until melted, about 3 minutes.

5. Remove from heat and serve immediately.

CARBS IN BELL PEPPERS

Bell peppers aren't the lowest-carb vegetable out there (a cup of chopped red bell pepper contains 6 grams of net carbs), but the nutrient trade-off is worth it. That same cup of bell pepper contains 190 milligrams of vitamin C—that's almost three times the amount you need for the entire day. Vitamin C boosts your immune system, fights inflammation, and keeps your bones and muscles strong. All bell peppers are a worthwhile part of a keto diet; just watch your portion sizes.

WHITE CHICKEN CHILI

Serves 6

Beef is often the star of chili, but in this recipe, chicken gets its time to shine. If you want to raise the fat content a bit, you can use chicken thighs in place of the chicken breasts. You'll also get a deeper flavor.

INGREDIENTS

2 cups Kettle & Fire Classic Chicken Bone Broth

1½ teaspoons minced garlic

1 (4.5-ounce) can chopped green chiles

1 small jalapeño, seeded and diced

1 small white onion, peeled and minced

1 medium stalk celery, finely diced

2½ teaspoons ground cumin

1 teaspoon dried oregano

1½ pounds boneless, skinless chicken breasts

⅓ cup grass-fed heavy cream

6 ounces cream cheese, softened

1 teaspoon sea salt

½ teaspoon ground black pepper

1. Add broth, garlic, chiles, jalapeño, onion, celery, cumin, and oregano to a slow cooker. Stir to combine. Add chicken breasts.

2. Cook on low for 6 hours.

3. Remove chicken from slow cooker and shred with two forks. Return shredded chicken to the slow cooker.

4. Whisk together cream, cream cheese, salt, and pepper in a medium bowl. Stir the mixture into slow cooker until smooth.

5. Cook for another 30 minutes on low. Serve immediately.

SPINACH AND ARTICHOKE CHICKEN

Serves 6

Marinated artichokes are a great way to add some extra fiber to this chicken dish. Artichokes are also loaded with prebiotics, which help feed the good bacteria in your gut and keep you healthy.

NET CARBS
6g

Calories: 391
Fat: 23g
Sodium: 945mg
Carbohydrates: 9g
Fiber: 3g
Sugar: 4g
Sugar alcohols: 0g
Protein: 37g

INGREDIENTS

1 teaspoon garlic powder

1 teaspoon onion powder

1 teaspoon sea salt

½ teaspoon ground black pepper

1½ pounds boneless, skinless chicken breasts, cubed

¼ cup Kettle & Fire Classic Chicken Bone Broth

1 (10-ounce) package frozen chopped spinach, thawed and squeezed dry

1 (14.5-ounce) jar marinated artichoke hearts, drained and chopped

8 ounces cream cheese, softened and cubed

½ cup shredded Parmesan cheese

¾ cup shredded whole milk mozzarella cheese

1. Combine garlic powder, onion powder, salt, and pepper in a large bowl. Add chicken cubes and toss to combine. Place chicken in slow cooker. Add chicken bone broth.

2. Cook on low for 4 hours. Add spinach, artichokes, cream cheese, and Parmesan cheese. Cook on low for an additional hour. Sprinkle mozzarella cheese on top and cover until cheese is melted, about 3 minutes.

3. Turn off heat and allow to cool for 5 minutes, then serve warm.

FIBER-RICH ARTICHOKES

Artichokes don't get a lot of attention, but they're low-carb nutritional powerhouses that deserve a chance in the spotlight. Artichokes are packed with antioxidants, and they're a good source of vitamin C, vitamin K, folate, and fiber. In fact, one medium artichoke has more fiber than a cup of prunes and only 12 grams of carbohydrates, a whopping 8 of which come from the fiber.

GARLIC-CRUSTED CHICKEN THIGHS

NET CARBS
3g

Calories: 358
Fat: 21g
Sodium: 577mg
Carbohydrates: 3g
Fiber: 0g
Sugar: 1g
Sugar alcohols: 0g
Protein: 36g

Serves 4

This recipe calls for garlic powder, but if you're a real garlic lover and want to kick it up a notch, add a teaspoon of minced garlic (in addition to the garlic powder) to the mixture before you coat the chicken.

INGREDIENTS

½ cup Tessemae's Organic Mayonnaise

½ cup Tessemae's Organic Habanero Ranch Dressing

¾ cup crushed EPIC Artisanal Sea Salt & Pepper Pork Rinds

1 teaspoon paprika

1 teaspoon garlic powder

1 pound boneless, skinless chicken thighs

1. Preheat oven to 375°F. Line a baking sheet with parchment paper and set aside.

2. Combine mayonnaise and ranch dressing in a small bowl and whisk until smooth.

3. In a shallow dish, combine pork rinds, paprika, and garlic powder.

4. Dip each chicken thigh in mayonnaise mixture, covering both sides, and press into pork rind mixture, coating entire chicken thigh.

5. Transfer thighs to prepared baking sheet.

6. Bake for 30 minutes or until juices run clear.

7. Remove from oven and serve immediately.

HEALTH BENEFITS OF GARLIC

Garlic is often regarded for its mouthwatering flavor, but there's a lot of nutrition packed into those little cloves as well. Studies show that garlic can help prevent and reduce inflammation, fight off certain cancers, and improve your blood pressure. Garlic also has strong antibacterial properties, so it may be able to help kill any potentially harmful bacteria that's lurking in your food.

SPICY SALSA CHICKEN

Serves 6

If you want to raise the fat content of this recipe a little bit, you can use chicken thighs in place of chicken breasts. Serve with Mexican-style cauliflower rice and a dollop of good-quality sour cream.

INGREDIENTS

2 teaspoons ground cumin

2 teaspoons chili powder

½ teaspoon paprika

½ teaspoon sea salt

¼ teaspoon ground black pepper

6 (4-ounce) boneless, skinless chicken breasts

1 (8-ounce) jar no-sugar-added hot salsa

½ cup canned no-sugar-added tomato sauce

2 teaspoons minced garlic

1 small red onion, peeled and diced

1. Combine cumin, chili powder, paprika, salt, and pepper in a small bowl. Sprinkle over chicken, coating all sides as much as possible.

2. Place chicken breasts in slow cooker. Pour salsa and tomato sauce on top. Add garlic and onion and cover.

3. Cook on low for 4 hours or until chicken is tender. Shred chicken with two forks and stir to combine.

4. Serve hot.

CHAPTER 6

BEEF, PORK, AND LAMB

STUFFED PORK TENDERLOIN

Serves 4

Pork is so versatile that you can use this recipe as a basic template and change the fillings to anything you want. For example, try ham instead of prosciutto or Gorgonzola cheese instead of feta.

NET CARBS
2g

Calories: 390
Fat: 27g
Sodium: 898mg
Carbohydrates: 3g
Fiber: 1g
Sugar: 1g
Sugar alcohols: 0g
Protein: 33g

INGREDIENTS

1 pound pork tenderloin

4 (0.5-ounce) slices prosciutto

4 slices Applegate Naturals No Sugar Bacon, cooked and chopped

½ teaspoon garlic powder

½ teaspoon ground sage

½ teaspoon ground black pepper

¼ teaspoon sea salt

½ teaspoon dry mustard

2 ounces cream cheese, softened

¼ cup crumbled feta cheese

1 cup frozen spinach, thawed and drained

3 tablespoons olive oil

1. Preheat oven to 350°F.

2. Butterfly pork tenderloin and set aside.

3. Lay each slice of prosciutto down on the pork.

4. Put bacon, garlic powder, sage, pepper, salt, mustard, cream cheese, feta cheese, and spinach in a medium bowl and beat with a handheld electric mixer on medium speed until smooth.

5. Spread filling over prosciutto and roll tenderloin closed. Secure pork with kitchen string.

6. Heat olive oil in a large skillet over medium-high heat. Sear pork for 2 minutes on each side, then place in an ungreased baking dish.

7. Bake for 30 minutes or until internal temperature reaches 160°F.

8. Remove from oven and allow to rest for 10 minutes, then slice and serve.

GRILLED LAMB BURGERS

Serves 4

If you want to make these burgers in the oven instead of on a grill, bake them at 325°F for about 35 minutes or until the lamb is cooked through. Make sure to watch them carefully as they cook so they don't dry out.

Calories: 240
Fat: 16g
Sodium: 582mg
Carbohydrates: 2g
Fiber: 0g
Sugar: 1g
Sugar alcohols: 0g
Protein: 19g

INGREDIENTS

1 pound ground lamb

1 teaspoon dried rosemary

1 teaspoon dried thyme

2 teaspoons minced garlic

½ teaspoon onion powder

½ teaspoon sea salt

½ teaspoon ground black pepper

2 tablespoons Tessemae's Organic Mayonnaise

2 tablespoons Dijon mustard

1 tablespoon Tessemae's Unsweetened Ketchup

1. Preheat grill to medium heat.

2. Combine lamb, rosemary, thyme, garlic, onion powder, salt, and pepper in a large bowl and mix thoroughly. Form into four equal-sized patties.

3. Cook on grill for 5 minutes on each side or until burgers reach desired level of doneness. Remove from heat and allow to rest for 5 minutes.

4. Whisk together mayonnaise, Dijon mustard, and ketchup in a small bowl, and spread on top of burgers before serving.

PHILLY CHEESESTEAK BAKE

Serves 6

The ground beef in this recipe is really easy to work with, but you can also use flank steak or other small steak strips if you prefer with no change to the carbohydrate count.

NET CARBS
5g

Calories: 487
Fat: 37g
Sodium: 855mg
Carbohydrates: 6g
Fiber: 1g
Sugar: 3g
Sugar alcohols: 0g
Protein: 32g

INGREDIENTS

1 tablespoon olive oil

1½ pounds 85/15 ground beef

1 tablespoon McCormick Grill Mates Montreal Steak Seasoning

1 teaspoon sea salt

½ teaspoon ground black pepper

½ cup minced green bell pepper

1 medium yellow onion, peeled and diced

2 teaspoons minced garlic

4 ounces cream cheese, softened

1 teaspoon coconut aminos

2 large eggs

½ cup grass-fed heavy cream

½ cup shredded Parmesan cheese

6 (1-ounce) slices provolone cheese

1. Preheat oven to 350°F.

2. Heat olive oil in a large skillet over medium heat. Crumble beef into skillet and cook until it starts to brown, about 2 minutes. Add steak seasoning, salt, black pepper, bell pepper, onion, and garlic, and continue cooking until beef is no longer pink, about 6 more minutes.

3. Stir in cream cheese and coconut aminos, and continue cooking until cream cheese is melted, about 2 minutes.

4. Transfer to an ungreased 6" × 9" casserole dish.

5. Whisk together eggs, cream, and Parmesan cheese in a separate medium bowl. Pour over beef mixture and stir to combine. Top with provolone cheese slices.

6. Bake for 20 minutes or until hot and bubbly. Remove from oven and allow to cool for 5 minutes, then serve warm.

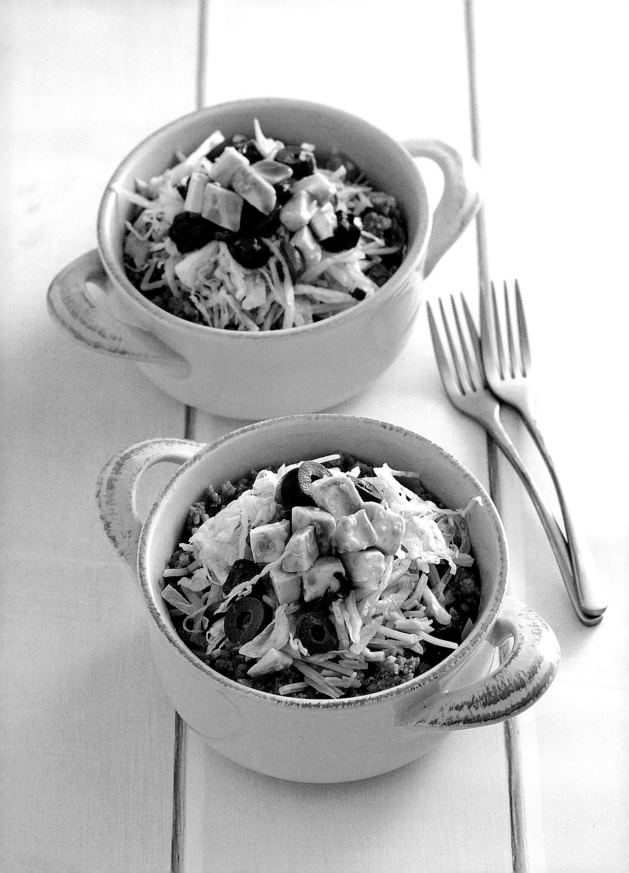

SPICY SAUSAGE BURRITO BOWLS

Serves 4

Instead of buying ground pork and seasoning it yourself, you can use premade spicy sausage as long as there isn't any added sugar in the ingredient list. Keep in mind that added sugar can go by several names, like brown sugar, honey, high-fructose corn syrup, or molasses.

Calories: 406
Fat: 31g
Sodium: 843mg
Carbohydrates: 6g
Fiber: 2g
Sugar: 2g
Sugar alcohols: 0g
Protein: 25g

INGREDIENTS

1 pound ground pork

1 teaspoon sea salt

1½ teaspoons ground sage

½ teaspoon ground black pepper

½ teaspoon crushed red pepper flakes

1 tablespoon olive oil

½ cup shredded Cheddar cheese

4 cups shredded iceberg lettuce

¼ cup chopped black olives

¼ cup sour cream

½ cup chopped avocado

4 teaspoons Cholula Original Hot Sauce

1. Combine pork, salt, sage, black pepper, and red pepper flakes in a large bowl and mix with your hands to evenly incorporate spices into meat.

2. Heat olive oil in a large skillet over medium heat and crumble pork into skillet. Cook until pork is no longer pink, about 8 minutes. Drain excess fat and divide evenly among four bowls.

3. Top each bowl with 2 tablespoons cheese, 1 cup lettuce, 1 tablespoon olives, 1 tablespoon sour cream, 2 tablespoons avocado, and 1 teaspoon hot sauce.

4. Serve immediately.

ITALIAN BEEF SKILLET

Serves 6

Rao's Homemade Marinara Sauce is one of the lowest-carbohydrate options out there, but you can use any jarred marinara sauce that doesn't have any added sugar. You can also make your own if you have the time, but make sure you factor in any change in carbs.

INGREDIENTS

1 tablespoon olive oil

2 cups riced cauliflower

1 small yellow onion, peeled and diced

1 teaspoon minced garlic

1½ pounds 85/15 ground beef

1 teaspoon sea salt

½ teaspoon ground black pepper

⅛ teaspoon crushed red pepper flakes

2 cups Rao's Homemade Marinara Sauce

½ cup Kettle & Fire Classic Beef Bone Broth

1 teaspoon Italian seasoning

2 cups shredded whole milk mozzarella cheese

¼ cup grated Parmesan cheese

1. Position oven rack on top of oven. Preheat broiler on high.

2. Heat olive oil in a large cast-iron skillet over medium heat. (If you don't have cast iron, you can use any ovenproof skillet.) Add cauliflower and cook until softened, about 5 minutes. Stir in onion and cook for another 2 minutes. Add garlic and cook until fragrant, about 30 seconds.

3. Crumble ground beef into skillet and sprinkle salt, black pepper, and red pepper flakes on top. Cook until beef is no longer pink, about 8 minutes.

4. Stir in marinara sauce, broth, and Italian seasoning. Reduce heat to low and simmer for 20 minutes or until sauce thickens.

5. Sprinkle cheeses on top and broil for 4 minutes or until cheese is hot and bubbly.

6. Remove from oven and allow to cool for 5 minutes, then serve warm.

STEAK TIPS WITH GRAVY

Serves 4

When it comes to xanthan gum, a little goes a long way. When you're thickening liquids like gravy or soup, you need only ¼ to ½ teaspoon of xanthan gum.

NET CARBS
2g

Calories: 211
Fat: 10g
Sodium: 801mg
Carbohydrates: 2g
Fiber: 0g
Sugar: 0g
Sugar alcohols: 0g
Protein: 28g

INGREDIENTS

For the steak tips:

1 tablespoon olive oil

1 pound sirloin steak tips

1 teaspoon garlic powder

½ teaspoon sea salt

¼ teaspoon ground black pepper

For the gravy:

2 cups Kettle & Fire Classic Beef Bone Broth

¼ teaspoon xanthan gum

½ cup sliced baby bella mushrooms

2 teaspoons salted grass-fed butter

1 teaspoon garlic powder

½ teaspoon sea salt

¼ teaspoon ground black pepper

1. To make the steak tips, heat olive oil in a large skillet over medium heat. Add steak tips to skillet and sprinkle evenly with garlic powder, salt, and pepper. Cook, stirring occasionally, until beef is browned on all sides, about 5 minutes.

2. To make the gravy, combine broth and xanthan gum in a separate small saucepan over low heat and stir until dissolved. Pour over meat.

3. Stir in mushrooms, butter, garlic powder, salt, and pepper. Cover, reduce heat to low, and simmer for 45 minutes or until gravy thickens.

4. Remove from heat and serve immediately.

WHAT IS XANTHAN GUM?

Xanthan gum, which is made from a fermentation process involving the bacterium Xanthomonas campestris, sounds like a scary additive that you should avoid—but it's actually a really handy keto thickener that's not known to have any serious ill effects in adults. In fact, xanthan gum can contribute to good health by increasing the amount of short-chain fatty acids (or SCFAs) in your gut. Although it can cause diarrhea if consumed in excess, most people tolerate normal amounts well. You shouldn't give xanthan gum to infants under the age of one.

ROPA VIEJA

Serves 6

Ropa vieja is one of the national dishes of Cuba, but it's also a staple in other areas of the world, like Puerto Rico and the Caribbean. Ropa vieja is usually served with rice, but you can mimic the traditional presentation and keep the dish keto-friendly by serving it with some steamed cauliflower rice.

NET CARBS
5g

Calories: 234
Fat: 14g
Sodium: 511mg
Carbohydrates: 6g
Fiber: 1g
Sugar: 3g
Sugar alcohols: 0g
Protein: 22g

INGREDIENTS

2 tablespoons olive oil, divided

1½ pounds flank steak

1 cup Kettle & Fire Classic Beef Bone Broth

1 (8-ounce) can no-sugar-added tomato sauce

1 small yellow onion, peeled and diced

1 small green bell pepper, seeded and sliced into strips

2 teaspoons minced garlic

2 tablespoons tomato paste

1½ teaspoons ground cumin

2 teaspoons sazón seasoning

½ teaspoon dried cilantro

1 tablespoon white vinegar

1. Heat 1 tablespoon olive oil in a large skillet over medium-high heat. Add steak and brown on each side.

2. Transfer to a slow cooker. Add remaining ingredients and stir until incorporated. Cover and cook on low for 8 hours.

3. Remove meat from slow cooker and shred with two forks. Serve immediately.

SPICY SAUSAGE AND ESCAROLE SOUP

NET CARBS
6g

Serves 6

This recipe has a kick, especially if you use the homemade sausage spice blend. If you want to dial it down a notch, reduce or omit the crushed red pepper. If you don't have a pressure cooker, you can make it in a slow cooker instead by cooking on low for 4 hours.

Calories: 217
Fat: 13g
Sodium: 924mg
Carbohydrates: 9g
Fiber: 3g
Sugar: 2g
Sugar alcohols: 0g
Protein: 16g

INGREDIENTS

1 tablespoon olive oil

1 large yellow onion, peeled and diced

2 tablespoons minced garlic

1 pound no-sugar-added pork sausage

4½ cups Kettle & Fire Classic Chicken Bone Broth

¼ cup chopped fresh parsley

1 large bunch escarole, coarsely chopped

1 teaspoon sea salt

1 teaspoon ground black pepper

½ teaspoon crushed red pepper flakes

1. Turn on the sauté function of your pressure cooker and add olive oil to the pot. Add onion and garlic and cook until softened, about 4 minutes. Add sausage and cook until no longer pink, about 7 minutes.

2. Add remaining ingredients to pot and stir to combine. Cover and make sure vent is closed.

3. Turn pressure cooker to soup function and set for 20 minutes. Start cook time.

4. When timer goes off, allow pressure to release naturally.

5. When pressure is released, remove pressure cooker lid and allow to cool for 5 minutes, then serve.

PORK SAUSAGE BLEND

Sometimes it can be difficult to find pork sausage without any added sugar or undesirable ingredients. To make your own, combine 1 teaspoon sea salt, ½ teaspoon dried parsley, ¼ teaspoon ground sage, ¼ teaspoon ground black pepper, ¼ teaspoon dried thyme, ¼ teaspoon crushed red pepper flakes, ⅛ teaspoon cayenne pepper, and ¼ teaspoon ground coriander in a small bowl. Mix into a pound of ground pork thoroughly before cooking.

SHEPHERD'S PIE

Serves 6

This recipe freezes very well, so save yourself some time down the road by doubling the recipe and freezing half for later. You can thaw and cook the frozen pie for dinner on a night that you don't feel like cooking.

Calories: 439
Fat: 34g
Sodium: 596mg
Carbohydrates: 9g
Fiber: 3g
Sugar: 3g
Sugar alcohols: 0g
Protein: 25g

INGREDIENTS

2 tablespoons coconut oil

1 medium yellow onion, peeled and chopped

3 cloves garlic, peeled and minced

2 medium stalks celery, diced

1 medium zucchini, diced

1½ pounds ground lamb

1 teaspoon dried rosemary

1 teaspoon dried thyme

1 teaspoon ground black pepper

½ teaspoon sea salt

½ teaspoon garlic powder

4 cups cauliflower florets, boiled until tender

¼ cup grass-fed heavy cream

3 tablespoons salted grass-fed butter

½ teaspoon garlic salt

¾ cup shredded Cheddar cheese

1. Preheat oven to 350°F.

2. Heat coconut oil in a large skillet over medium-high heat. Add onion and garlic and sauté until softened, about 5 minutes. Add celery and zucchini and sauté for another 5 minutes.

3. Add lamb, rosemary, thyme, pepper, salt, and garlic powder, and cook until lamb is no longer pink, about 7 minutes. Transfer lamb mixture to an ungreased 9" × 13" baking dish.

4. Put boiled cauliflower, cream, butter, and garlic salt in a food processor, and pulse until smooth. Pour cauliflower mixture on top of lamb. Top with cheese.

5. Bake until cheese is melted and pie is bubbly, about 25 minutes. Remove from oven and allow to cool for 10 minutes, then serve.

THE HISTORY OF SHEPHERD'S PIE

Shepherd's pie was first developed in an attempt to use up leftover meat. Traditional shepherd's pie uses lamb. When beef is used instead of lamb, the same meal is called cottage pie.

ROASTED LEG OF LAMB

Serves 8

If you can't find an 8-pound leg of lamb at your grocery store, call your local butcher or meat shop and make a special order. You may have to wait a few days, but it will be worth it.

Calories: 700
Fat: 44g
Sodium: 708mg
Carbohydrates: 2g
Fiber: 1g
Sugar: 0g
Sugar alcohols: 0g
Protein: 69g

INGREDIENTS

1 (8-pound) whole leg of lamb

1 teaspoon sea salt

½ teaspoon ground black pepper

⅔ cup yellow mustard

1 tablespoon Worcestershire sauce

2 teaspoons minced garlic

½ teaspoon dried thyme

½ teaspoon dried rosemary

½ teaspoon dried basil

1. Preheat oven to 325°F.

2. Place lamb in an ungreased roasting pan and sprinkle with salt and pepper.

3. Combine remaining ingredients in a small bowl and mix well.

4. Spread mustard mixture all over lamb, coating evenly.

5. Roast for 2½ hours or until lamb reaches an internal temperature of 145°F. Remove from oven and allow to rest for 10 minutes, then slice and serve.

BEEF CARNITAS

Serves 6

Beef Carnitas is the perfect foundation for a homemade, keto-friendly burrito bowl.

Calories: 334
Fat: 21g
Sodium: 568mg
Carbohydrates: 2g
Fiber: 1g
Sugar: 0g
Sugar alcohols: 0g
Protein: 33g

INGREDIENTS

2 pounds chuck roast

1 tablespoon chili powder

½ teaspoon dried oregano

½ teaspoon ground cumin

½ (4-ounce) can diced green chiles

1½ teaspoons minced garlic

1 teaspoon sea salt

2 cups Kettle & Fire Classic Beef Bone Broth

3 medium fresh jalapeños, seeded and minced

1. Season chuck roast with spices. Transfer to a slow cooker.

2. Add remaining ingredients, cover, and cook on low for 6 hours or until beef reaches an internal temperature of 160°F.

3. Remove meat from slow cooker and shred with two forks. Return to slow cooker and stir.

4. Cook for another 30 minutes. Cool for 5 minutes, then serve warm.

CHEESEBURGER MEATLOAF

Serves 6

When assembling this meatloaf, make sure you pinch the bottom and top halves together to form a tight seal. If you don't, the cheese will leak out of the sides. The finished product will still be delicious, but it'll be a lot messier too!

NET CARBS
4g

Calories: 496
Fat: 30g
Sodium: 1,318mg
Carbohydrates: 4g
Fiber: 0g
Sugar: 2g
Sugar alcohols: 0g
Protein: 49g

INGREDIENTS

For the meatloaf:

1½ pounds 85/15 ground beef

1 cup crushed EPIC Oven Baked Pink Himalayan and Sea Salt Pork Rinds

1 large egg, lightly beaten

1 tablespoon Worcestershire sauce

2 tablespoons Tessemae's Unsweetened Ketchup

1 teaspoon onion powder

1 teaspoon dried minced onion

1 teaspoon garlic powder

1 teaspoon sea salt

8 ounces sharp Cheddar cheese, cut into cubes

For the sauce:

¼ cup Tessemae's Organic Mayonnaise

2 tablespoons Tessemae's Unsweetened Ketchup

1 tablespoon dill pickle juice

1 tablespoon minced dill pickle

1 tablespoon yellow mustard

½ teaspoon onion powder

½ teaspoon garlic powder

1. Preheat oven to 350°F.

2. To make the meatloaf, combine beef, pork rinds, egg, Worcestershire sauce, ketchup, onion powder, minced onion, garlic powder, and salt in a large bowl. Use your hands to mix ingredients until fully incorporated.

3. Arrange half of the beef mixture in an ungreased 9" × 5" loaf pan and press down, making an even layer. Use your hands to form an indentation in the meat and press cheese cubes evenly into it.

4. Press the rest of the beef mixture on top, making sure to form a seal where the two halves meet.

5. Bake for 55 minutes or until hot and bubbly and meat reaches an internal temperature of 160°F.

6. While meatloaf is cooking, make the sauce by combining all sauce ingredients in a small bowl. Whisk until smooth.

7. Remove meatloaf from oven and allow to rest for 10 minutes. Top meatloaf with sauce and serve.

LAMB CHOPS WITH MINT BUTTER

Serves 6

Make sure to rub the butter on the lamb chops while they're still hot from the grill. This helps ensure that the flavor from the butter covers the lamb chops completely.

INGREDIENTS

For the mint butter:

½ cup salted grass-fed butter, softened

2 tablespoons chopped fresh mint

2 tablespoons chopped fresh basil

1 teaspoon minced garlic

⅛ teaspoon ground black pepper

For the lamb chops:

3 tablespoons olive oil

12 (4-ounce) lamb chops

1½ teaspoons sea salt

1 teaspoon ground black pepper

1. Preheat grill to high heat.

2. To make the mint butter, combine mint butter ingredients in a medium bowl and beat with a handheld electric mixer on medium speed until smooth. Set aside.

3. To make the lamb chops, brush olive oil evenly on both sides of each chop. Sprinkle with salt and pepper.

4. Cook on the preheated grill for 2½ minutes on each side or until lamb chops reach desired level of doneness.

5. Remove from heat and rub equal parts mint butter on each lamb chop while still hot.

6. Serve immediately.

PAPRIKA PORK SKILLET

Serves 6

If the paprika you have in your spice cabinet doesn't have an additional qualifier, it's likely sweet paprika. While many dishes that call for paprika are flexible, this one really shines with the sweeter flavor.

Calories: 240
Fat: 14g
Sodium: 497mg
Carbohydrates: 4g
Fiber: 1g
Sugar: 2g
Sugar alcohols: 0g
Protein: 24g

INGREDIENTS

2 tablespoons sweet paprika, divided

1 teaspoon sea salt

½ teaspoon ground black pepper

1½ pounds pork loin, cut into cubes

2 tablespoons olive oil

1 small yellow onion, peeled and diced

2 teaspoons minced garlic

1 teaspoon dried thyme

½ cup diced tomatoes

½ cup Kettle & Fire Classic Chicken Bone Broth

½ cup sour cream

1. Combine 1 tablespoon paprika, salt, and pepper in a large bowl and mix well. Add pork to bowl and toss to coat evenly. Set aside.

2. Heat olive oil in a large skillet over medium heat. Add onion and cook until softened, about 3 minutes. Add garlic, remaining paprika, and thyme, and cook for 3 minutes.

3. Stir in pork and cook until no longer pink, about 8 minutes. Add tomatoes and broth and stir.

4. Reduce heat to low and simmer for 10 minutes. Remove from heat and stir in sour cream.

5. Allow to cool for 5 minutes, then serve warm.

THE THREE TYPES OF PAPRIKA

There are three types of paprika: sweet, smoked, and hot. While they're all perfectly acceptable for a keto diet, they do have different taste profiles. Sweet paprika has a sweet pepper flavor, with little to no spice. Smoked paprika, also called Spanish paprika, is made from smoked peppers and has a richer, smoky flavor that's similar to what you'd find in smoked bacon. Hot paprika is spicy and has a peppery taste. If a recipe calls for hot paprika and you don't have any on hand, you can mimic the flavor by combining sweet paprika with a dash of cayenne pepper.

PIZZA MEATBALLS

Serves 6 (Makes 24 meatballs)

These Pizza Meatballs are like mini pizzas on the go. They're easy to take with you and delicious cold, so they're the perfect option for when you have to take your meals to work or somewhere that you might not have access to a stove or microwave to reheat them.

NET CARBS

6g

Calories: 532
Fat: 40g
Sodium: 1,468mg
Carbohydrates: 6g
Fiber: 0g
Sugar: 4g
Sugar alcohols: 0g
Protein: 36g

INGREDIENTS

1½ pounds ground meatloaf mix

¼ cup chopped fresh parsley

1 teaspoon dried oregano

1 teaspoon dried basil

1 large egg, lightly beaten

1 teaspoon minced garlic

1 teaspoon sea salt

1 (28-ounce) jar Rao's Homemade Marinara Sauce

¾ cup chopped no-sugar-added pepperoni

1 cup shredded whole milk mozzarella cheese

1 cup shredded provolone cheese

1. Grease the inside of a slow cooker with olive oil cooking spray.

2. Combine meatloaf mix, parsley, oregano, basil, egg, garlic, and salt in a medium bowl. Mix with hands until fully incorporated.

3. Shape mixture into twenty-four equal-sized meatballs and place meatballs in the bottom of the prepared slow cooker.

4. Pour sauce on top of meatballs and add chopped pepperoni. Cover and cook on low for 5 hours or until meatballs are cooked through.

5. Sprinkle cheeses on top, cover, and continue cooking on low for another 30 minutes.

6. Allow meatballs to cool for 5 minutes, then serve warm.

LAMB MEATBALLS

Serves 6 (Makes 24 meatballs)

Lamb and mint are two flavors that complement each other really well, but if mint isn't your thing, you can swap it out for some more fresh parsley for equally delicious results.

NET CARBS

4g

Calories: 373
Fat: 29g
Sodium: 628mg
Carbohydrates: 5g
Fiber: 1g
Sugar: 2g
Sugar alcohols: 0g
Protein: 23g

INGREDIENTS

For the meatballs:

1½ pounds ground lamb

1 teaspoon minced garlic

1 teaspoon sea salt

½ teaspoon ground black pepper

1 teaspoon chopped fresh mint

2 tablespoons chopped fresh parsley

¼ cup finely crumbled feta cheese

¼ cup almond flour

1 large egg, lightly beaten

For the sauce:

1 cup sour cream

1½ tablespoons olive oil

1 tablespoon fresh lemon juice

1½ tablespoons chopped fresh mint

½ teaspoon minced garlic

¼ teaspoon sea salt

1 small cucumber, peeled and grated

1. Preheat oven to 375°F. Line two baking sheets with parchment paper and set aside.

2. To make the meatballs, combine meatball ingredients in a large bowl and use your hands to mix together.

3. Scoop mixture up by the tablespoon and form into twenty-four equal-sized meatballs. Arrange on prepared baking sheets.

4. Bake for 20 minutes or until lamb is cooked through.

5. While meatballs are cooking, make the sauce by combining all sauce ingredients, except cucumber, in a food processor. Pulse until smooth. Transfer to a small bowl and stir in cucumber.

6. Remove meatballs from oven and allow to cool for 5 minutes, then serve warm with dipping sauce.

EGG ROLL SKILLET

Serves 6

This recipe combines all of the best flavors of an egg roll but ditches the carbs that come from the egg roll wrapper. You can eat it on its own or serve it with a side of cauliflower fried rice.

INGREDIENTS

2 tablespoons sesame oil

½ cup diced yellow onion

6 green onions, trimmed and chopped, white and green parts separated

1 teaspoon minced garlic

1½ pounds 85/15 ground beef

1 tablespoon Wildbrine Spicy Kimchi Sriracha sauce

1 tablespoon Worcestershire sauce

2 teaspoons minced fresh ginger

¼ teaspoon ground black pepper

3 cups shredded Napa cabbage

2 tablespoons coconut aminos

1 tablespoon apple cider vinegar

1. Heat sesame oil in a large skillet over medium-high heat. Add yellow onion and white parts of green onions. Cook until softened, about 5 minutes. Add garlic and cook for another 30 seconds.

2. Crumble beef into skillet and cook for 2 minutes. Stir in sriracha, Worcestershire sauce, ginger, and pepper. Cook until beef is no longer pink, about 6 more minutes.

3. Add remaining ingredients except green parts of green onions, stir, and cover until cabbage is tender, about 8 minutes. Remove from heat, stir, and top with green parts of green onions.

4. Serve immediately.

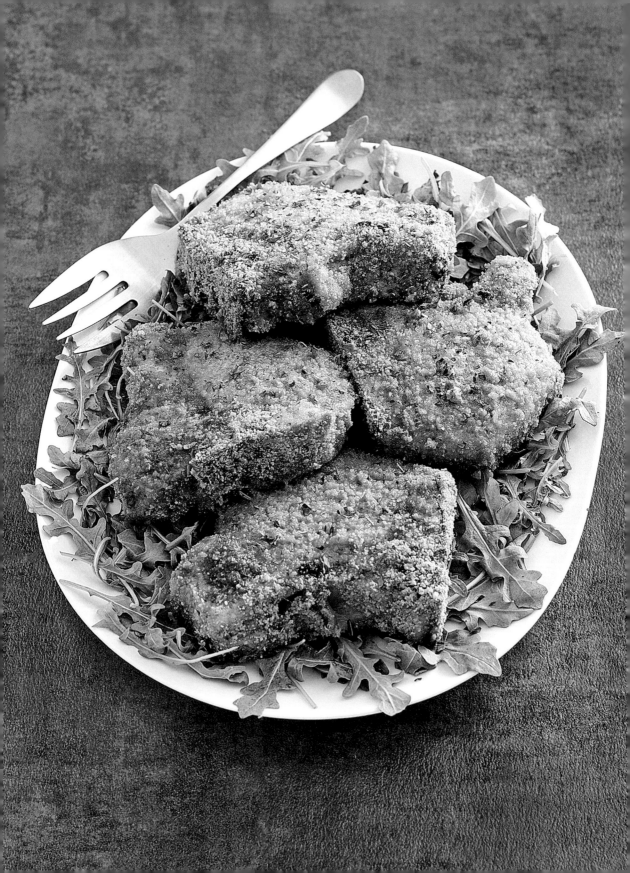

PARMESAN-CRUSTED PORK CHOPS

Serves 4

If you don't have pork rinds, you can use coarse almond meal in their place. You'll lose some crispiness (and add a few carbs), but still end up with a delicious, keto-friendly breading. Nutrition-packed arugula is a great addition to the meal.

NET CARBS
2g

Calories: 426
Fat: 22g
Sodium: 726mg
Carbohydrates: 2g
Fiber: 0g
Sugar: 0g
Sugar alcohols: 0g
Protein: 51g

INGREDIENTS

2 large eggs

1½ cups crushed EPIC Oven Baked Pink Himalayan and Sea Salt Pork Rinds

½ cup grated Parmesan cheese

1½ teaspoons dried parsley

1½ teaspoons garlic powder

1 teaspoon onion powder

4 (4-ounce) pork chops

1. Preheat oven to 400°F. Line a baking sheet with parchment paper and set aside.

2. Add eggs to a medium bowl and whisk lightly. Set aside.

3. Combine remaining ingredients except pork chops in a shallow dish and mix well.

4. Dip each pork chop into the eggs and then press into pork rind mixture, coating both sides evenly.

5. Arrange on the prepared baking sheet and bake for 15 minutes or until pork reaches an internal temperature of 145°F.

6. Remove from oven and allow to cool for 5 minutes, then serve warm.

BUTTER STEAK WITH GARLIC AND CHIVES

NET CARBS
1g

Serves 4

Adding the butter to the steak after cooking not only adds a load of healthy fats, but it also creates a soft texture that makes this steak melt in your mouth. If you don't have access to an outdoor grill, you can cook the steak in a skillet over medium heat instead.

Calories: 294
Fat: 22g
Sodium: 631mg
Carbohydrates: 1g
Fiber: 0g
Sugar: 0g
Sugar alcohols: 0g
Protein: 23g

INGREDIENTS

1 tablespoon avocado oil

4 tablespoons unsalted grass-fed butter, softened

2 teaspoons minced garlic

2 teaspoons chopped fresh chives

1 teaspoon sea salt

½ teaspoon ground black pepper

4 (4-ounce) filet mignon steaks

1. Preheat grill to high heat. Brush avocado oil on grill grate.

2. Combine butter, garlic, and chives in a small bowl, and stir to mix well.

3. Sprinkle salt and pepper on both sides of steaks. Place steaks on preheated grill and cook for 5 minutes on each side or until steaks reach desired level of doneness.

4. Remove steaks from grill and brush with butter mixture. Loosely cover with foil and allow to rest for 10 minutes, then serve warm.

BEEF CURRY

Serves 6

Garam masala is an Indian-inspired spice blend that combines cumin, coriander, cardamom, and cinnamon (among other things). If you don't have any premixed garam masala, you can easily make your own at home with spices that you probably already have in your cabinet (see the following sidebar).

NET CARBS
3g

Calories: 360
Fat: 23g
Sodium: 513mg
Carbohydrates: 4g
Fiber: 1g
Sugar: 2g
Sugar alcohols: 0g
Protein: 33g

INGREDIENTS

2 tablespoons olive oil

1 small yellow onion, peeled and diced

1½ pounds 85/15 ground beef

1 large tomato, seeded and diced

1 tablespoon curry powder

1 teaspoon garam masala

1½ teaspoons paprika

1 teaspoon sea salt

½ teaspoon ground black pepper

¼ teaspoon cayenne pepper

½ cup Kettle & Fire Classic Beef Bone Broth

3 tablespoons sour cream

1. Heat olive oil in a large skillet over medium heat. Add onion and cook until softened, about 5 minutes. Crumble beef into skillet and cook until no longer pink, about 8 minutes. Drain excess fat.

2. Stir in tomato and spices and reduce heat to low. Cook until tomato releases its juices, about 10 minutes.

3. Add broth and simmer for 30 minutes. Remove from heat and stir in sour cream.

4. Allow to cool for 5 minutes, then serve warm.

HOMEMADE GARAM MASALA

To make your own garam masala, combine 1 tablespoon ground cumin, 1½ teaspoons ground coriander, 1½ teaspoons ground cardamom, 1½ teaspoons ground black pepper, 1 teaspoon ground cinnamon, ½ teaspoon ground cloves, and ½ teaspoon ground nutmeg, and mix well. You can use what you need and then store the rest in an airtight container in your pantry for up to 6 months.

CHAPTER 7

SEAFOOD

BLACKENED TUNA STEAKS

Serves 4

Like any great blackened dish, this tuna has a little kick. If it's too spicy for you, scale back on the cayenne pepper or omit it completely.

NET CARBS
5g

Calories: 377
Fat: 26g
Sodium: 1,213mg
Carbohydrates: 7g
Fiber: 2g
Sugar: 1g
Sugar alcohols: 0g
Protein: 28g

INGREDIENTS

2 tablespoons olive oil

2 tablespoons fresh lime juice

1 tablespoon minced garlic

4 (4-ounce) tuna steaks

2 tablespoons paprika

1 teaspoon cayenne pepper

1 tablespoon onion powder

1 tablespoon garlic powder

2 teaspoons sea salt

1 teaspoon ground black pepper

1 teaspoon dried basil

1 teaspoon dried oregano

¼ cup Nutiva Organic Coconut Oil with Buttery Flavor

1. Combine olive oil, lime juice, and minced garlic in a large resealable bag. Add tuna steaks to bag, seal, and toss to coat. Refrigerate for 2 hours.

2. Mix paprika, cayenne pepper, onion powder, garlic powder, salt, black pepper, basil, and oregano together in a small bowl.

3. Remove tuna steaks from marinade and completely coat each side with spice mixture.

4. Heat coconut oil in a large skillet over medium heat. Add coated tuna steaks to the skillet and cook for 4 minutes on each side.

5. Remove from heat and serve immediately.

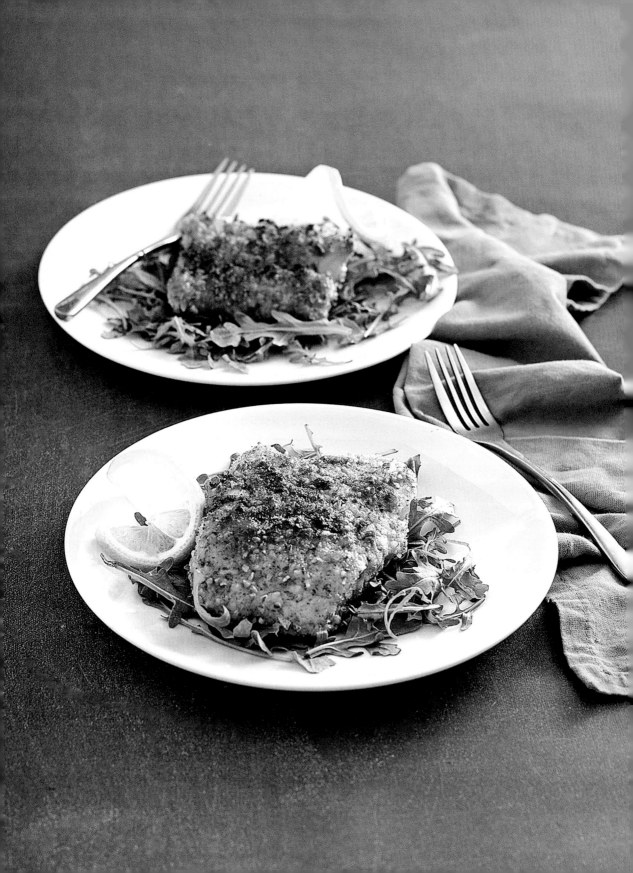

ALMOND-COATED HALIBUT

Serves 6

If you have some extra time, you can make your own halibut breading by starting out with whole raw almonds and pulsing them until a thick crumb forms. This will create a crunchier crust than you'll get with pre-ground almond meal, but it is more time-consuming. Serve atop a bed of arugula.

INGREDIENTS

¼ cup coarse almond meal

1 teaspoon sea salt

½ teaspoon ground black pepper

1 teaspoon McCormick Old Bay Seasoning

½ cup finely minced almonds

2 large eggs

6 (4-ounce) halibut fillets

¼ cup unsalted grass-fed butter, melted

1. Position oven rack in the middle of your oven. Preheat broiler on high. Line a baking sheet with parchment paper and set aside.

2. Combine almond meal, salt, pepper, Old Bay seasoning, and minced almonds in a shallow dish. Mix well.

3. Add eggs to a medium bowl and whisk lightly. Dip each fillet in eggs and then press into almond mixture, coating both sides evenly. Place coated fillets on prepared baking sheet and pour melted butter on top.

4. Broil for 6 minutes or until fish flakes easily with a fork.

5. Remove from oven and serve immediately.

PARMESAN-CRUSTED COD

Serves 4

McCormick Old Bay Seasoning is a combination of paprika, celery salt, and dry mustard that complements any fish dish perfectly. If you don't have any, you can make your own using the recipe in the following sidebar.

NET CARBS 1g

Calories: 162
Fat: 8g
Sodium: 215mg
Carbohydrates: 1g
Fiber: 0g
Sugar: 0g
Sugar alcohols: 0g
Protein: 20g

INGREDIENTS

¼ cup grated Parmesan cheese

2 tablespoons salted grass-fed butter, softened

1 tablespoon Tessemae's Organic Mayonnaise

½ teaspoon onion powder

½ teaspoon dried parsley

½ teaspoon paprika

¼ teaspoon ground black pepper

¼ teaspoon garlic salt

4 (4-ounce) cod fillets

1 teaspoon McCormick Old Bay Seasoning

1. Preheat broiler on high. Position oven rack in the middle of your oven. Line a broiler pan with aluminum foil and spray with cooking spray.

2. In a small bowl, combine cheese, butter, mayonnaise, onion powder, parsley, paprika, pepper, and garlic salt. Set aside.

3. Arrange cod fillets on broiler pan and sprinkle with Old Bay seasoning. Broil fish for 2 minutes, flip each fillet, and then broil for another 2 minutes.

4. Remove fish from oven and spread cheese mixture evenly on top of each fillet.

5. Return to the oven and broil for another 2 minutes or until fish flakes easily with a fork.

6. Remove from oven and serve immediately.

MAKING YOUR OWN FISH SEASONING

If you don't have McCormick Old Bay Seasoning, you can make your own copycat version by combining 2 tablespoons celery salt, ½ teaspoon paprika, ¼ teaspoon ground black pepper, ¼ teaspoon cayenne pepper, ⅛ teaspoon dry mustard, ⅛ teaspoon ground nutmeg, ⅛ teaspoon ground cinnamon, ⅛ teaspoon ground cardamom, ⅛ teaspoon allspice, ⅛ teaspoon ground cloves, and ⅛ teaspoon ground ginger. Use what you need and then store the rest in an airtight container in your spice cabinet for up to 6 months.

SPICY SCALLOPS

Serves 6

When it comes to scallops, timing is everything. They don't take long to cook and can overcook quickly if you don't watch the clock. When scallops are browned on both sides and break apart along the edge, they're done. Serve over spaghetti squash or zucchini noodles.

INGREDIENTS

- 1 tablespoon salted grass-fed butter
- 1 tablespoon minced garlic
- 2 cups grass-fed heavy cream
- 1 teaspoon dried basil
- 1 teaspoon dried thyme
- 2 teaspoons sea salt
- 1 teaspoon ground black pepper
- 1 teaspoon ground white pepper
- 1 teaspoon crushed red pepper flakes
- ½ teaspoon Cajun seasoning
- 1 cup chopped green onions
- 1 cup chopped fresh parsley
- 1½ pounds bay scallops
- ½ cup shredded whole milk mozzarella cheese
- ½ cup grated Parmesan cheese

1. Heat butter in a large deep skillet over medium heat. Add garlic and cook for 1 minute. Stir in cream and bring to a simmer, whisking constantly. Don't let the cream boil.

2. When the cream starts to simmer, reduce heat to low and stir in basil, thyme, salt, black pepper, white pepper, red pepper flakes, Cajun seasoning, green onions, and parsley. Simmer for 7 minutes, whisking frequently, until thickened.

3. Add scallops and cook for 6 minutes. Stir in cheeses until smooth.

4. Remove from heat and serve.

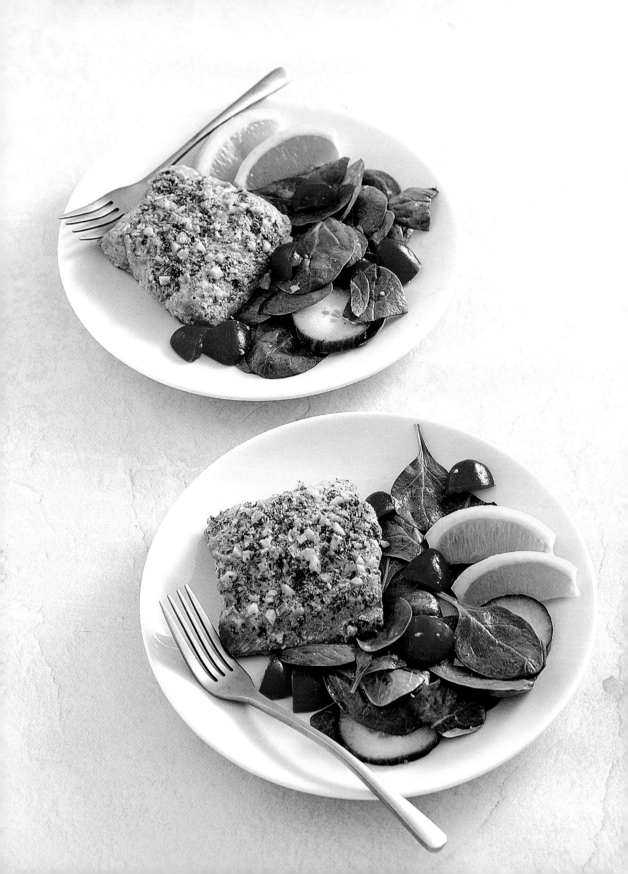

BAKED LEMON GARLIC SALMON

Serves 4

This Baked Lemon Garlic Salmon is almost completely devoid of carbs and loaded with healthy omega-3 fatty acids that help fight inflammation and keep your brain sharp. Serve with Breadless Broccoli Gratin (see recipe in Chapter 9) or a side salad.

Calories: 338
Fat: 26g
Sodium: 640mg
Carbohydrates: 2g
Fiber: 0g
Sugar: 0g
Sugar alcohols: 0g
Protein: 23g

INGREDIENTS

- 1 tablespoon minced garlic
- ¼ cup olive oil
- 3 tablespoons unsalted grass-fed butter, melted
- 1 teaspoon dried basil
- 1 teaspoon sea salt
- 1 teaspoon ground black pepper
- 3 tablespoons fresh lemon juice
- 1 teaspoon dried parsley
- 4 (4-ounce) wild Alaskan salmon fillets, skin removed

1. Combine all ingredients except salmon in a large resealable plastic bag. Add salmon fillets to the bag and seal. Massage the oil mixture into the salmon and then refrigerate for 1 hour.

2. Preheat oven to 375°F.

3. Transfer salmon fillets to an ungreased 9" × 13" baking dish and pour marinade on top.

4. Bake for 30 minutes or until salmon flakes easily with a fork.

5. Remove from oven and serve immediately.

DECADENT CRAB CAKES

Serves 2 (Makes 4 crab cakes)

Crab cakes sound really fancy, but they come together in a matter of minutes. Serve them on top of a salad or with your favorite side dish from Chapter 9 to make them a complete meal.

NET CARBS
4g

Calories: 452
Fat: 33g
Sodium: 2,022mg
Carbohydrates: 8g
Fiber: 4g
Sugar: 2g
Sugar alcohols: 0g
Protein: 32g

INGREDIENTS

2 (6-ounce) cans wild-caught lump crabmeat, drained

2 tablespoons Tessemae's Organic Mayonnaise

2 large eggs, lightly beaten

¼ cup minced red bell pepper

½ cup coarse almond meal

2 tablespoons fresh lime juice

1 teaspoon sea salt

3 tablespoons chopped fresh parsley

2 teaspoons Frank's RedHot Original Cayenne Pepper Sauce

2 tablespoons avocado oil

1. Combine all ingredients except avocado oil in a medium bowl and mix until combined.

2. Form into four equal-sized patties.

3. Heat avocado oil in a medium skillet over medium-high heat. Add patties and cook for 3 minutes, flip over, and cook for an additional 3 minutes or until golden brown.

4. Remove from heat and serve.

CRAB-TOPPED COD

Serves 6

Although this recipe calls for cod, you can use any mild-flavored whitefish with equally delicious results—and without much change to the net carb count.

Calories: 262
Fat: 16g
Sodium: 548mg
Carbohydrates: 2g
Fiber: 0g
Sugar: 1g
Sugar alcohols: 0g
Protein: 28g

INGREDIENTS

6 (4-ounce) cod fillets, skin removed

6 tablespoons unsalted grass-fed butter, divided

½ teaspoon sea salt

½ teaspoon ground black pepper

1 medium stalk celery, minced

¼ cup minced red bell pepper

2 tablespoons minced shallots

1 teaspoon minced garlic

1 (6-ounce) can wild-caught lump crabmeat, drained

¼ cup crushed EPIC Oven Baked Pink Himalayan and Sea Salt Pork Rinds

1 large egg, lightly beaten

½ cup grated Parmesan cheese

2 tablespoons fresh lemon juice

1. Preheat oven to 350°F.

2. Arrange cod fillets in an ungreased 9" × 13" baking dish. Melt 4 tablespoons butter and brush on top of each fillet. Sprinkle fillets evenly with salt and pepper and cover. Bake for 20 minutes.

3. While fish is baking, heat remaining butter in a large skillet over medium heat.

4. Add celery, bell pepper, shallots, and garlic, and cook until celery and pepper are softened, about 5 minutes. Remove from heat and stir in remaining ingredients.

5. Top each fillet with crab mixture, cover, and return to the oven for 10 minutes.

6. Remove from oven and serve immediately.

SALMON-STUFFED AVOCADO

NET CARBS
3g

Calories: 298
Fat: 21g
Sodium: 504mg
Carbohydrates: 10g
Fiber: 7g
Sugar: 1g
Sugar alcohols: 0g
Protein: 21g

Serves 4

This Salmon-Stuffed Avocado recipe combines a large dose of omega-3 fatty acids from the salmon with loads of monounsaturated fats from the avocado, making it as healthy and satiating as it is delicious. This recipe is also a great way to use up any leftover salmon you may have from a previous night's dinner.

INGREDIENTS

2 large avocados

2 cups canned wild Alaskan pink salmon, drained

¼ cup peeled and diced cucumber

2 tablespoons Tessemae's Pantry Classic Ranch Dressing & Marinade

1 teaspoon minced red onion

1 teaspoon dried parsley

¼ teaspoon sea salt

¼ teaspoon ground black pepper

¼ teaspoon paprika

⅛ teaspoon onion powder

⅛ teaspoon garlic powder

1. Slice avocados in half lengthwise and remove the pit. Scoop out 1 tablespoon avocado flesh from each avocado half and transfer to a medium bowl. Set avocado halves aside.

2. Mash avocado flesh and add remaining ingredients to bowl. Stir to incorporate.

3. Scoop equal amounts salmon mixture into each avocado half and serve immediately.

DIJON SALMON FILLETS

Serves 4

Most bottled mustards—including Dijon and regular yellow—are free of carbohydrates, but double-check the ingredient lists and nutrition facts before purchasing. Some flavored mustards may have added sugar.

Calories: 287
Fat: 19g
Sodium: 563mg
Carbohydrates: 2g
Fiber: 1g
Sugar: 0g
Sugar alcohols: 0g
Protein: 24g

INGREDIENTS

4 (4-ounce) skin-on wild Alaskan salmon fillets

¼ cup Dijon mustard

¼ teaspoon sea salt

¼ teaspoon ground black pepper

¼ cup coarse almond meal

½ teaspoon dried basil

¼ teaspoon dried oregano

¼ teaspoon dried thyme

⅛ teaspoon garlic powder

¼ cup unsalted grass-fed butter

1. Preheat oven to 400°F. Line a baking sheet with parchment paper and set aside.

2. Arrange salmon, skin side down, on prepared baking sheet.

3. Spread 1 tablespoon mustard on top of each fillet and sprinkle evenly with salt and pepper. Set aside.

4. Combine almond meal, basil, oregano, thyme, and garlic powder in a small bowl, and mix well.

5. Heat butter in a small saucepan on low heat. When butter is melted, add almond meal mixture and stir to incorporate. Spoon almond meal mixture evenly on top of each fillet.

6. Bake for 15 minutes, then turn broiler to low. Broil for 2 minutes, watching closely, or until almond topping crisps.

7. Remove from oven and serve immediately.

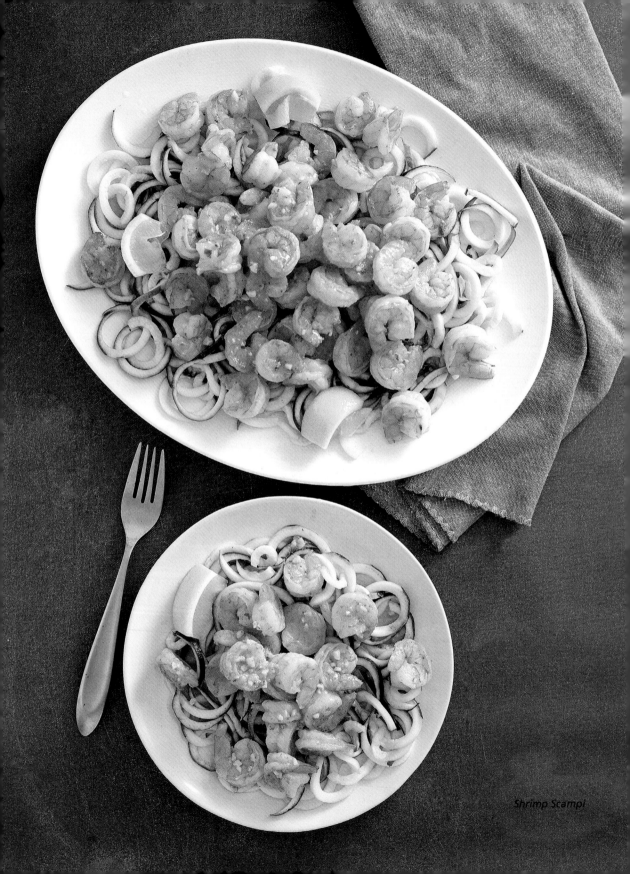

Shrimp Scampi

SHRIMP SCAMPI

Serves 4

NET CARBS
1g

This dish is easy to prepare and extremely versatile. Pour it over zucchini noodles or a plate of spinach. If you have room in your daily macros for some extra carbohydrates, try spooning it over spaghetti squash.

Calories: 421
Fat: 35g
Sodium: 131mg
Carbohydrates: 1g
Fiber: 0g
Sugar: 0g
Sugar alcohols: 0g
Protein: 28g

INGREDIENTS

¾ cup unsalted grass-fed butter

2 cloves garlic, peeled and minced

1 tablespoon fresh lemon juice

1 pound cooked medium shrimp, shelled, deveined, and tails removed

1. Melt butter in a large skillet over medium heat. When butter is hot, add garlic and sauté until translucent, about 4 minutes.

2. Add lemon juice and shrimp and cook over medium heat until shrimp is hot, about 2 minutes.

3. Remove from heat and serve shrimp with garlic butter poured on top.

CRAB ENDIVE CUPS

Serves 2 (Makes 4 endive cups)

NET CARBS
1g

These Crab Endive Cups highlight the rich flavor of the crab by adding only simple ingredients.

Calories: 95
Fat: 8g
Sodium: 242mg
Carbohydrates: 2g
Fiber: 1g
Sugar: 0g
Sugar alcohols: 0g
Protein: 3g

INGREDIENTS

¼ cup canned wild-caught lump crabmeat, drained

2 tablespoons avocado flesh

1 teaspoon finely chopped fresh cilantro

1 tablespoon chopped green onion

1 teaspoon fresh lime juice

1 tablespoon coconut oil

⅛ teaspoon sea salt

⅛ teaspoon ground black pepper

4 Belgian endive leaves, washed and dried

1. Add all ingredients except endive to a small food processor. Pulse to mix until well blended.

2. Divide crab mixture evenly among endive leaves.

3. Serve immediately.

SPICY CAJUN COD

Serves 4

This Spicy Cajun Cod combines red pepper flakes, cayenne pepper, and paprika to give you a mouthwatering kick. If you want to dial back the spice, reduce the amount of Cajun seasoning and replace with garlic powder, onion powder, and paprika.

NET CARBS

2g

Calories: 165
Fat: 9g
Sodium: 208mg
Carbohydrates: 2g
Fiber: 0g
Sugar: 1g
Sugar alcohols: 0g
Protein: 18g

INGREDIENTS

1 tablespoon Cajun seasoning

½ teaspoon lemon pepper

¼ teaspoon sea salt

¼ teaspoon ground black pepper

4 (4-ounce) cod fillets

3 tablespoons unsalted grass-fed butter

2 tablespoons fresh lemon juice

2 tablespoons minced shallots

1. Combine Cajun seasoning, lemon pepper, salt, and black pepper in a small bowl and mix well.

2. Sprinkle seasoning mixture equally on both sides of each cod fillet.

3. Heat butter in a large skillet over medium-high heat. Add lemon juice and shallots and cook for 1 minute.

4. Add cod fillets and cook for 3 minutes, spooning butter mixture on top of cod while it's cooking. Turn fillets over and cook for another 3 minutes or until fish flakes easily with a fork.

5. Remove from heat and allow to rest for 2 minutes, then serve warm.

LEMON DILL SALMON

Serves 4

This recipe calls for dried dill since it's already a part of many spice cabinets, but you can use fresh dill weed. For every 1 teaspoon dried dill, substitute 1 tablespoon fresh dill.

NET CARBS
2g

Calories: 242
Fat: 16g
Sodium: 203mg
Carbohydrates: 2g
Fiber: 0g
Sugar: 0g
Sugar alcohols: 0g
Protein: 23g

INGREDIENTS

4 (4-ounce) wild Alaskan salmon fillets, skin removed

¼ cup unsalted grass-fed butter

2 teaspoons minced garlic

2 teaspoons dried or 2 tablespoons fresh chopped dill

¼ cup fresh lemon juice

¼ teaspoon sea salt

¼ teaspoon ground black pepper

8 thin lemon slices

1. Preheat oven to 350°F. Cut four squares of aluminum foil, each about twice the size of a salmon fillet, and place on a baking sheet. Arrange each salmon fillet on top of each aluminum foil square.

2. Heat butter in a small saucepan over low heat. Add garlic and dill and cook for 2 minutes. Remove from heat and stir in lemon juice.

3. Pour equal parts butter mixture on top of each salmon fillet. Sprinkle with salt and pepper. Arrange 2 lemon slices on top of each salmon fillet.

4. Wrap aluminum foil around each fillet and bake for 20 minutes or until salmon flakes easily with a fork.

5. Remove from oven and serve immediately.

SALMON PICCATA

Serves 2

NET CARBS
5g

If you don't have herbes de Provence seasoning, you can season this sauce with rosemary, thyme, basil, marjoram, oregano, tarragon, parsley, or any combination of dried or fresh herbs that you like. The amount of capers may seem minimal, but don't skip them! They add a nice saltiness and some antioxidants to the dish.

Calories: 362
Fat: 25g
Sodium: 1,597mg
Carbohydrates: 6g
Fiber: 1g
Sugar: 0g
Sugar alcohols: 0g
Protein: 28g

INGREDIENTS

1 teaspoon sea salt

½ teaspoon ground black pepper

2 (4-ounce) wild Alaskan salmon fillets, skin removed

½ cup water

2 tablespoons unsalted grass-fed butter

1 tablespoon minced garlic

1 cup Kettle & Fire Classic Chicken Bone Broth

½ teaspoon xanthan gum

¼ cup Native Forest Organic Heavy Coconut Cream

2 tablespoons fresh lemon juice

1 teaspoon herbes de Provence seasoning

¼ teaspoon dried minced onion

2 tablespoons capers

1. Sprinkle salt and pepper on salmon and set salmon on top of a trivet in your pressure cooker. Add water to the pot.

2. Secure the lid and cook on the steam setting for 15 minutes.

3. While salmon is cooking, add butter and garlic to a medium skillet over medium heat. Cook for 4 minutes or until garlic starts to turn golden brown. Add broth, xanthan gum, coconut cream, lemon juice, herb seasoning, onion, and capers to the skillet. Stir to combine.

4. Reduce heat to low and continue cooking until sauce thickens, about 5 minutes, stirring frequently.

5. When salmon is done cooking, allow pressure to release naturally. Remove lid and transfer salmon fillets to a plate. Spoon sauce on top. Serve hot.

PAN-FRIED FISH STICKS

Serves 4

NET CARBS
3g

Calories: 379
Fat: 28g
Sodium: 189mg
Carbohydrates: 6g
Fiber: 3g
Sugar: 1g
Sugar alcohols: 0g
Protein: 26g

You can also make these fish sticks in an air fryer by spraying the battered sticks with some avocado or olive oil cooking spray and then air-frying them at 375°F for 15 to 20 minutes, turning once during cooking. Either way, these fish sticks cook quickly for an easy weeknight meal.

INGREDIENTS

1 cup coarse almond meal

1 teaspoon McCormick Old Bay Seasoning

⅛ teaspoon sea salt

⅛ teaspoon ground black pepper

2 large eggs

1 pound boneless cod fillets, cut into 1" strips

¼ cup Nutiva Organic Coconut Oil with Buttery Flavor, divided

1. Combine almond meal, Old Bay seasoning, salt, and pepper in a shallow dish and mix well. Set aside.

2. Add eggs to a small bowl and whisk lightly. Dip each cod strip into egg and then press into almond meal mixture, coating each side completely.

3. Heat 2 tablespoons coconut oil in a large skillet over medium heat. Add half of the cod strips to the pan and cook for 3 minutes on each side. Remove cod and place on a paper towel–lined plate.

4. Wipe skillet clean and heat remaining coconut oil over medium heat and repeat with remaining cod strips.

5. Remove from heat and serve immediately.

SPINACH AND FETA– STUFFED SWORDFISH

Serves 4

This stuffed swordfish looks fancy, but it comes together quickly with ingredients that you probably already have on hand. Make sure you're using mature spinach, which has more texture and holds up to cooking better than baby spinach.

Calories: 262
Fat: 17g
Sodium: 271mg
Carbohydrates: 3g
Fiber: 1g
Sugar: 1g
Sugar alcohols: 0g
Protein: 23g

INGREDIENTS

4 (4-ounce) swordfish steaks

2 tablespoons olive oil, divided

1 tablespoon fresh lemon juice

2 teaspoons minced garlic

½ cup chopped white mushrooms

3 cups chopped fresh spinach

½ cup crumbled feta

1. Preheat broiler on high. Position oven rack in the middle of your oven. Line a baking sheet with parchment paper and set aside.

2. Cut a slit into each swordfish steak to create a pocket. Arrange swordfish on prepared baking sheet.

3. Combine 1 tablespoon olive oil and lemon juice in a small bowl. Brush the mixture on both sides of each swordfish steak.

4. Heat remaining olive oil in a large skillet over medium heat. Add garlic and cook for 1 minute. Add mushrooms and cook until they start to soften, about 3 minutes. Stir in spinach and cook until wilted, about 3 more minutes.

5. Add feta and stir to incorporate. Cook for 1 more minute and remove from heat.

6. Stuff equal parts of spinach mixture into the slit of each swordfish steak.

7. Broil for 12 minutes or until fish flakes easily with a fork. Remove from broiler and serve immediately.

EASY GRILLED SHRIMP

Serves 6

NET CARBS
3g

If you don't have access to a grill, you can make this shrimp in the oven by pouring the shrimp and the marinade (after it marinates for 30 minutes) in a baking dish and baking the shrimp at 350°F for about 10 minutes. Serve with Herb-Roasted Asparagus or Jalapeño Popper Mashed Cauliflower (see recipes in Chapter 9).

Calories: 406
Fat: 37g
Sodium: 1,184mg
Carbohydrates: 3g
Fiber: 0g
Sugar: 1g
Sugar alcohols: 0g
Protein: 16g

INGREDIENTS

1 cup olive oil

¼ cup chopped fresh parsley

3 tablespoons fresh lemon juice

½ teaspoon lemon zest

2 tablespoons Frank's RedHot Original Cayenne Pepper Sauce

2 teaspoons minced garlic

1 tablespoon Tessemae's Unsweetened Ketchup

2 teaspoons herbes de Provence

1 teaspoon sea salt

1 teaspoon ground black pepper

⅛ teaspoon cayenne pepper

1½ pounds large shrimp, peeled and deveined

1. Combine all ingredients, except shrimp, in a large resealable plastic bag. Shake to combine.

2. Add shrimp and reseal. Massage to coat shrimp with marinade and refrigerate for 30 minutes.

3. Preheat grill to medium-low heat. Cover grilling tray with aluminum foil.

4. Transfer shrimp and marinade to prepared grilling tray.

5. Grill shrimp, turning once during cooking, until shrimp turns opaque, about 10 minutes.

6. Remove from heat and serve immediately.

BENEFITS OF SHRIMP

Shrimp is an unusually concentrated source of the carotenoid astaxanthin, which acts as an antioxidant and an anti-inflammatory agent. Shrimp is also an excellent source of the mineral selenium, which helps keep your thyroid hormones in balance.

LEMON SALMON BURGERS

NET CARBS
4g

Serves 4

These burgers call for canned salmon, but make sure it's the wild Alaskan salmon. Wild-caught fish is significantly more nutritious and less contaminated than farm-raised fish.

Calories: 313
Fat: 22g
Sodium: 755mg
Carbohydrates: 5g
Fiber: 1g
Sugar: 2g
Sugar alcohols: 0g
Protein: 25g

INGREDIENTS

3 (6-ounce) cans wild Alaskan pink salmon, drained

2 large eggs, lightly beaten

¼ cup chopped fresh parsley

2 tablespoons minced white onion

¼ cup coarse almond meal

½ teaspoon Italian seasoning

2 tablespoons fresh lemon juice

¼ teaspoon sea salt

¼ teaspoon ground black pepper

⅛ teaspoon crushed red pepper flakes

½ cup Tessemae's Organic Habanero Ranch Dressing

1. Preheat oven to 325°F. Line a baking sheet with parchment paper and set aside.

2. Combine all ingredients except ranch dressing in a medium bowl and mix just until incorporated. Form into four equal-sized patties and arrange patties on prepared baking sheet.

3. Bake for 10 minutes, flip burgers over, then bake for an additional 10 minutes.

4. Remove from oven and serve each burger with 2 tablespoons ranch dressing.

GO WILD

Wild-caught fish is not only more nutritious than its farmed-raised counterpart, but it also contains significantly fewer toxins. According to reports, farm-raised salmon contains almost ten times more polychlorinated biphenyls (PCBs) than wild salmon. PCBs are toxins that increase the risk of stroke, insulin resistance, obesity, and diabetes. It's also higher in dioxins, a toxin that's been linked to heart disease, infertility, and hormonal issues.

152   200 UNDER 20g NET CARBS

COD AU GRATIN

Serves 4

This recipe calls for cod, but the basic cheese sauce is a keto-friendly accompaniment to any whitefish or chicken. If you want to incorporate some variety without significantly affecting the carb count, you can use haddock or 1 pound boneless, skinless chicken breasts in place of the cod. Of course, you'll have to adjust the cooking time to about 40 minutes for the chicken.

NET CARBS
6g

Calories: 641
Fat: 56g
Sodium: 1,095mg
Carbohydrates: 7g
Fiber: 1g
Sugar: 4g
Sugar alcohols: 0g
Protein: 28g

INGREDIENTS

4 (4-ounce) cod fillets

1¼ teaspoons sea salt, divided

¼ teaspoon ground black pepper

3 tablespoons unsalted grass-fed butter

1 teaspoon minced garlic

¼ cup minced shallots

1 tablespoon yellow mustard

½ teaspoon McCormick Old Bay Seasoning

1½ cups grass-fed heavy cream

2 ounces cream cheese

1 cup shredded white Cheddar cheese

½ teaspoon paprika

1. Preheat oven to 350°F.

2. Arrange cod fillets in an ungreased 8" × 8" baking dish and sprinkle with 1 teaspoon salt and pepper.

3. Melt butter in a medium saucepan over medium heat. Add garlic and cook for 1 minute. Add shallots and cook for another 2 minutes. Stir in remaining salt, mustard, Old Bay seasoning, and heavy cream, and cook for 7 minutes or until thickened, stirring constantly.

4. Add cream cheese and stir until melted. Stir in Cheddar cheese until smooth.

5. Pour sauce over cod and sprinkle with paprika.

6. Bake for 30 minutes or until gratin is bubbling and fish is cooked through.

7. Remove from oven and allow to cool for 5 minutes, then serve warm.

MARGHERITA HADDOCK FILLETS

NET CARBS
3g

Calories: 219
Fat: 11g
Sodium: 702mg
Carbohydrates: 4g
Fiber: 1g
Sugar: 2g
Sugar alcohols: 0g
Protein: 25g

Serves 4

This simple, fresh dish is perfect for a weeknight when you want something satisfying and healthy, but without a lot of effort. For a richer flavor, try to use fresh mozzarella cheese instead of pre-packaged slices.

INGREDIENTS

4 (4-ounce) haddock fillets

½ teaspoon sea salt

¼ teaspoon ground black pepper

1 teaspoon minced garlic

1 medium tomato, seeded and diced

¼ cup minced yellow onion

4 teaspoons olive oil

2 teaspoons balsamic vinegar

4 (1-ounce) slices whole milk mozzarella cheese

½ cup chopped fresh basil

1. Preheat oven to 400°F.

2. Cut four aluminum foil squares, each about twice the size of a haddock fillet, and arrange on a baking sheet. Place one haddock fillet on the center of each square.

3. Sprinkle salt and pepper evenly on fillets. Top with equal amounts of garlic, tomato, and onion. Drizzle 1 teaspoon olive oil and ½ teaspoon balsamic vinegar on top of each fillet and cover with a slice of mozzarella cheese.

4. Wrap aluminum foil around each fillet and bake until fish flakes easily with a fork, about 15 minutes.

5. Remove from oven, open foil packets, and sprinkle fresh basil on top.

6. Serve immediately.

CHAPTER 8

MEATLESS FAVORITES

KALE AND EGGS

Serves 6

Adding leafy greens like kale to your breakfast is a great way to make sure you're optimizing the amount of nutrients you're taking in while cutting carbs. Baby kale is milder and more tender than the mature leaves, so it will blend nicely into these eggs.

NET CARBS
3g

Calories: 213
Fat: 15g
Sodium: 504mg
Carbohydrates: 4g
Fiber: 1g
Sugar: 1g
Sugar alcohols: 0g
Protein: 16g

INGREDIENTS

1 tablespoon salted grass-fed butter, melted

3 cups baby kale leaves

8 large eggs, lightly beaten

1½ cups shredded whole milk mozzarella cheese, divided

¼ cup sliced green onion

½ teaspoon sea salt

½ teaspoon ground black pepper

¼ teaspoon dried dill

¼ teaspoon dried parsley

¼ teaspoon garlic powder

⅛ teaspoon dry mustard

1. Preheat oven to 375°F. Spread butter evenly on the bottom of an 8" × 12" casserole dish.

2. Sprinkle kale evenly on top of butter.

3. Combine eggs, ½ cup cheese, green onion, salt, pepper, dill, parsley, garlic powder, and dry mustard in a large bowl, and whisk well. Pour on top of kale.

4. Sprinkle remaining cheese on top.

5. Bake for 30 minutes or until eggs are set and cheese starts to bubble and brown.

6. Remove from oven and allow to cool for 5 minutes, then serve warm.

ALL HAIL THE KALE

It's no secret that kale consistently tops the charts as one of the highest-rated superfoods. That's because kale packs in a ton of nutrients for almost no carbs or calories. A single cup of kale contains more vitamin A, vitamin C, and vitamin K than you need for the entire day, but contributes only 7 calories and 0.06 grams of net carbs (which is basically nothing). If you're not a huge fan of kale, try baby kale instead of the mature leaves. It's still packed with nutrition, but easier on the palate due to its mild taste.

MAPLE AND BROWN SUGAR PORRIDGE

NET CARBS

6g

Calories: 575
Fat: 48g
Sodium: 231mg
Carbohydrates: 34g
Fiber: 24g
Sugar: 3g
Sugar alcohols: 4g
Protein: 15g

Serves 2

This low-carb porridge mimics the feel and texture of oats, but it's even more filling. That's because unlike oats, which are loaded with carbs, it contains both healthy fats from the hemp hearts and filling protein and fiber from the chia seeds.

INGREDIENTS

½ cup grass-fed heavy cream

½ cup unsweetened vanilla almond milk

¼ cup hemp hearts

2 tablespoons chia seeds

2 tablespoons ground flaxseed meal

2 tablespoons unsweetened shredded coconut

¼ cup almond flour

2 tablespoons ChocZero Maple Syrup

2 teaspoons Swerve Brown sweetener

1 teaspoon salted grass-fed butter

⅛ teaspoon sea salt

1 teaspoon vanilla extract

1. Combine cream and almond milk in a small saucepan and heat over low heat. When mixture is hot, stir in hemp hearts, chia seeds, flaxseed, and coconut.

2. Add remaining ingredients and mix well.

3. Cook for 5 minutes or until thickened, stirring constantly.

4. Remove from heat and serve immediately.

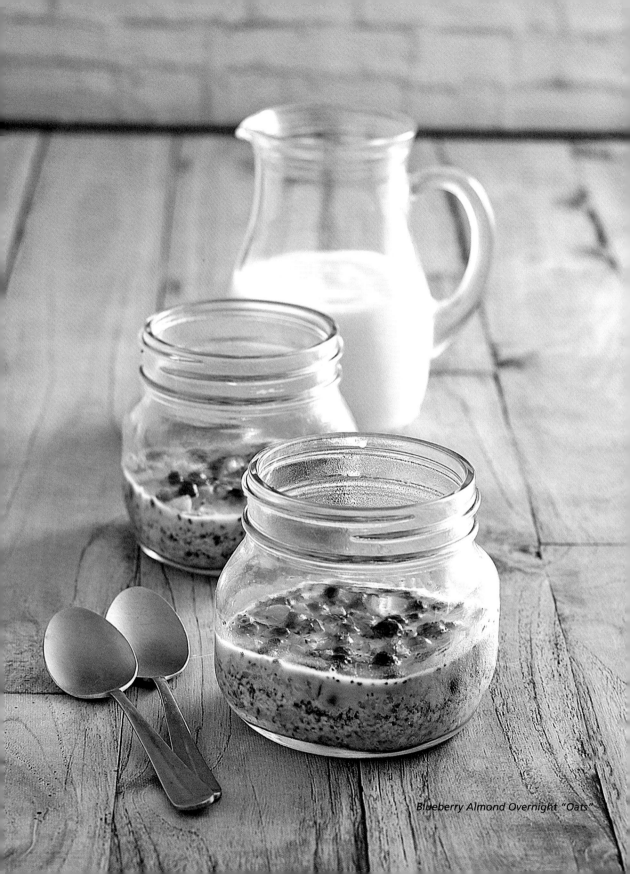

Blueberry Almond Overnight "Oats"

BLUEBERRY ALMOND OVERNIGHT "OATS"

NET CARBS
5g

Serves 2

While a small amount of blueberries is okay, be mindful of how much you add, because the carbs can add up quickly.

Calories: 326
Fat: 24g
Sodium: 163mg
Carbohydrates: 15g
Fiber: 10g
Sugar: 3g
Sugar alcohols: 0g
Protein: 16g

INGREDIENTS

⅔ cup full-fat coconut milk

½ cup hemp hearts

1 tablespoon chia seeds

2 teaspoons ChocZero Maple Syrup

¼ teaspoon vanilla extract

⅛ teaspoon almond extract

⅛ teaspoon sea salt

2 tablespoons crushed almonds

1 tablespoon frozen unsweetened wild blueberries

1. Combine all ingredients in a medium bowl and mix well.

2. Divide mixture in half and pour into two 16-ounce widemouthed Mason jars. Cover and refrigerate overnight. Serve cold.

CHOCOLATE BREAKFAST MILKSHAKE

NET CARBS
8g

Serves 2

This "milkshake" is made with good-for-you ingredients that won't spike your blood sugar and will keep you full until lunch.

Calories: 554
Fat: 53g
Sodium: 66mg
Carbohydrates: 22g
Fiber: 14g
Sugar: 6g
Sugar alcohols: 0g
Protein: 7g

INGREDIENTS

¾ cup full-fat coconut milk

¾ cup grass-fed heavy cream

1 tablespoon no-sugar-added almond butter

1 tablespoon raw cacao powder

1 tablespoon ChocZero Maple Syrup

⅔ cup frozen avocado pieces

2 scoops Perfect Keto Chocolate MCT Oil Powder

1. Combine all ingredients in a blender and blend until smooth.

2. Serve immediately.

GREEK-STYLE SPAGHETTI SQUASH PASTA

Serves 6

Calories: 131
Fat: 9g
Sodium: 273mg
Carbohydrates: 9g
Fiber: 2g
Sugar: 4g
Sugar alcohols: 0g
Protein: 4g

This Greek-Style Spaghetti Squash Pasta is an easy weeknight meal that takes almost no effort at all (once you get the spaghetti squash cut, of course). If you're extra hungry and want to add some plant-based protein, you can toss some hemp hearts into the mix.

INGREDIENTS

1 small spaghetti squash (should be about 4½ cups cooked)

1 tablespoon olive oil

1 tablespoon salted grass-fed butter

1 medium yellow onion, peeled and finely diced

½ cup chopped red bell pepper

2 teaspoons minced garlic

1 cup chopped grape tomatoes

⅔ cup crumbled feta cheese

¼ cup sliced kalamata olives

2 tablespoons chopped fresh basil

1. Preheat oven to 400°F. Line a baking sheet with parchment paper and set aside.

2. Arrange squash, cut side down, on baking sheet and bake for 45 minutes or until a fork can be easily inserted into the squash. Remove squash from oven and allow to cool for 5 minutes.

3. Heat olive oil and butter in a large skillet over medium heat. Add onion and bell pepper and cook until softened, about 5 minutes. Add garlic and cook for another minute.

4. Stir in tomatoes and cook until broken down, about 4 minutes. Stir in feta and olives.

5. Remove from heat and set aside.

6. Remove squash strands from cooked spaghetti squash and transfer to skillet with tomato mixture. Toss to coat.

7. Stir in basil, remove from heat, and serve.

MUSHROOM AND BLUE CHEESE SPAGHETTI SQUASH

NET CARBS
6g

Calories: 177
Fat: 14g
Sodium: 569mg
Carbohydrates: 8g
Fiber: 2g
Sugar: 4g
Sugar alcohols: 0g
Protein: 6g

Serves 6

Blue cheese has a distinctive taste that really helps bring out the mushroom in this dish, but if you prefer something milder, you can substitute soft goat cheese or some crumbled feta. If you use feta, you may want to reduce the added salt.

INGREDIENTS

1 tablespoon olive oil

1 small spaghetti squash (should be about 4½ cups cooked)

½ teaspoon garlic salt

½ teaspoon ground black pepper, divided

1 tablespoon salted grass-fed butter

1 large shallot, peeled and minced

8 ounces sliced baby bella mushrooms

2 teaspoons minced garlic

2 cups chopped fresh spinach

3 ounces cream cheese

2 tablespoons grass-fed heavy cream

½ teaspoon sea salt

½ cup crumbled blue cheese

1. Preheat oven to 400°F. Line a baking sheet with parchment paper and set aside.

2. Brush olive oil on flesh of spaghetti squash and sprinkle garlic salt and ¼ teaspoon pepper on top. Arrange on baking sheet, cut side down, and bake for 45 minutes or until a fork inserts easily into flesh. Remove from oven, but leave oven on.

3. While squash is cooling, heat butter in a medium skillet over medium heat. Add shallot and mushrooms and cook until mushrooms are tender, about 6 minutes. Stir in garlic and cook for another minute.

4. Add spinach and cook until wilted, about 3 minutes. Stir in cream cheese, heavy cream, salt, and remaining pepper. Continue cooking, stirring occasionally, until cream cheese is melted and ingredients are incorporated.

5. Use a fork to remove spaghetti squash strands from skin. Add squash to skillet and toss to coat. Cook for another 2 minutes.

6. Transfer squash to an ungreased 9" × 13" baking dish and top with blue cheese. Bake for 5 minutes or until cheese is melted and bubbly.

7. Remove from oven and allow to cool for 5 minutes, then serve warm.

EGGPLANT CASSEROLE

Serves 4

It's often called a vegetable, but eggplant is actually a berry, botanically speaking. But even though it's technically a fruit, eggplant is still low in carbs, providing only 2.3 grams of net carbs per cup.

INGREDIENTS

1 medium eggplant, peeled and diced

1¼ teaspoons sea salt, divided

2 teaspoons Italian seasoning

½ teaspoon ground black pepper

¼ teaspoon crushed red pepper flakes

1½ cups shredded sharp Cheddar cheese, divided

½ cup diced tomatoes

1 teaspoon minced garlic

1 large shallot, peeled and minced

1 large egg, lightly beaten

½ teaspoon dried parsley

1. Preheat oven to 350°F.

2. Place eggplant in a strainer over the sink and sprinkle with ¼ teaspoon salt. Let sit for 10 minutes to allow excess liquid to drain.

3. Transfer eggplant to a medium saucepan and cover with water. Bring to a boil, cover, and reduce heat to low.

4. Simmer for 7 minutes or until eggplant is tender. Drain and transfer cooked eggplant to an ungreased 1½-quart casserole dish.

5. Sprinkle remaining salt, Italian seasoning, black pepper, and red pepper flakes on top of eggplant and stir to combine.

6. Mix in ½ cup cheese, tomatoes, garlic, shallot, and egg. Sprinkle remaining cheese and parsley on top.

7. Bake for 30 minutes or until casserole is bubbling and cheese starts to brown. Remove from oven and allow to cool for 5 minutes, then serve warm.

ZOODLES WITH AVOCADO CREAM SAUCE

Serves 6

These zoodles require no cooking and are ready in 10 minutes flat. However, if you prefer your zoodles warm and slightly softened, you can sauté them in hot oil for a couple of minutes before tossing them with the sauce.

Calories: 248
Fat: 21g
Sodium: 22mg
Carbohydrates: 16g
Fiber: 9g
Sugar: 5g
Sugar alcohols: 0g
Protein: 6g

INGREDIENTS

3 cups fresh basil

1 cup water

⅓ cup pine nuts

¼ cup fresh lemon juice

½ teaspoon lemon zest

3 large avocados, peeled and pitted

3 large zucchini, spiralized

¾ cup halved cherry tomatoes

1. Combine basil, water, pine nuts, lemon juice, lemon zest, and avocados in a food processor or blender. Blend until smooth.

2. Place zucchini in a large bowl and pour avocado cream sauce on top. Toss to coat. Add tomatoes and toss to combine.

3. Serve immediately.

CAULIFLOWER RISOTTO

Serves 4

This low-carb version of risotto uses cauliflower instead, and the dish is so flavorful, you won't even know the difference!

Calories: 282
Fat: 25g
Sodium: 687mg
Carbohydrates: 8g
Fiber: 3g
Sugar: 3g
Sugar alcohols: 0g
Protein: 6g

INGREDIENTS

¼ cup unsalted grass-fed butter

1 large shallot, peeled and minced

1 teaspoon minced garlic

1 (12-ounce) bag riced cauliflower

⅔ cup sliced baby bella mushrooms

½ cup grass-fed heavy cream

½ cup grated Parmesan cheese

¾ teaspoon sea salt

½ teaspoon ground black pepper

¼ teaspoon ground nutmeg

⅛ teaspoon crushed red pepper flakes

1. Melt butter in a large skillet over medium heat. Add shallot and cook until softened, about 4 minutes. Stir in garlic and cook for another minute.

2. Add cauliflower and cook until just starting to soften, about 4 minutes. Stir in mushrooms and continue cooking for 4 more minutes.

3. Stir in remaining ingredients and cook until thick and creamy, about 5 minutes.

4. Remove from heat and serve immediately.

BAKED STUFFED PORTO-BELLO MUSHROOMS

NET CARBS
9g

Calories: 257
Fat: 19g
Sodium: 1,392mg
Carbohydrates: 13g
Fiber: 4g
Sugar: 7g
Sugar alcohols: 0g
Protein: 10g

Serves 2 (Makes 4 stuffed mushrooms)

Portobello mushrooms are a popular choice for meatless meals because they're thick and hearty and make you feel like you're eating a really substantial meal. In this dish, portobello mushrooms provide the base for a combination of low-carb vegetables and cheeses that will fill you up quickly.

INGREDIENTS

- 4 large portobello mushrooms, stems removed
- 2 tablespoons olive oil
- ½ cup chopped red bell pepper
- ¼ cup diced yellow onion
- 1 teaspoon minced garlic
- 1 teaspoon sea salt
- ½ teaspoon ground black pepper
- 2 tablespoons shredded Parmesan cheese
- 4 slices (about 1 ounce each) provolone cheese

1. Position oven rack in the center of the oven. Preheat oven to 350°F. Line a baking sheet with parchment paper and set aside.

2. Arrange mushrooms, stem side up, on prepared baking sheet.

3. Heat olive oil in a medium skillet over medium heat and add bell pepper and onion. Cook until softened, about 6 minutes. Stir in garlic and cook for another minute. Remove from heat and stir in salt, black pepper, and Parmesan cheese.

4. Scoop one-fourth of mixture into each mushroom cap. Top with a slice of provolone cheese.

5. Bake for 10 minutes. Turn broiler on high and broil for another 5 minutes or until cheese is browned and bubbly.

6. Remove from broiler and allow to cool for 5 minutes, then serve warm.

CAULIFLOWER MAC 'N' CHEESE

Serves 6

With this recipe, you no longer have to miss traditional macaroni and cheese when you're following a keto diet. If you want a more traditional pasta feel, replace the cauliflower with cooked spaghetti squash.

NET CARBS
6g

Calories: 286
Fat: 24g
Sodium: 647mg
Carbohydrates: 9g
Fiber: 3g
Sugar: 3g
Sugar alcohols: 0g
Protein: 11g

INGREDIENTS

2 tablespoons olive oil

1 teaspoon sea salt

½ teaspoon ground black pepper

¼ teaspoon garlic powder

1 teaspoon dried parsley

1 large head cauliflower, cut into bite-sized florets

1 cup shredded Cheddar cheese

½ cup shredded Gruyère cheese

½ cup grass-fed heavy cream

1 tablespoon salted grass-fed butter

⅛ teaspoon ground nutmeg

¼ cup grated Parmesan cheese

1. Preheat oven to 450°F. Line a baking sheet with parchment paper and set aside.

2. Combine olive oil, salt, pepper, garlic powder, and parsley in a medium bowl. Add cauliflower and toss to coat.

3. Arrange cauliflower on prepared baking sheet in a single layer. Roast 15 minutes or until browned and crispy. Transfer cauliflower to an ungreased 8" × 8" baking dish.

4. Combine remaining ingredients except Parmesan cheese in a medium saucepan over medium heat. Stir and allow to simmer for 5 minutes. Pour over cauliflower and toss to coat completely. Sprinkle Parmesan cheese on top.

5. Bake for 10 minutes or until cheese starts to brown. Remove from oven and allow to cool for 5 minutes, then serve warm

CAULI TIKKA MASALA

Serves 6

If you don't have xanthan gum, simply omit it and make the rest of the recipe as written. Xanthan gum will thicken the sauce a bit, but omitting it won't make a difference in the flavor.

INGREDIENTS

For the roasted cauliflower:

1 cup sour cream

1 tablespoon garam masala

1 tablespoon fresh lemon juice

1 teaspoon ground black pepper

1 teaspoon minced fresh ginger

1 large cauliflower head, cut into florets

For the tikka masala:

1 cup grass-fed heavy cream

¾ cup canned no-sugar-added tomato sauce

2 teaspoons minced garlic

1 tablespoon garam masala

½ teaspoon ground turmeric

½ teaspoon ground coriander

½ teaspoon sea salt

¼ teaspoon ground cinnamon

¼ teaspoon chili powder

¼ teaspoon xanthan gum

1. Preheat oven to 400°F. Line a baking sheet with parchment paper and set aside.

2. To make the roasted cauliflower, combine sour cream, 1 tablespoon garam masala, lemon juice, pepper, and ginger in a large bowl, and whisk well. Add cauliflower to bowl and toss to coat.

3. Arrange cauliflower in a single layer on prepared baking sheet and bake for 20 minutes.

4. While cauliflower is roasting, make the tikka masala: Combine tikka masala ingredients in a large skillet over medium heat. Bring to a simmer, then reduce heat to low.

5. Simmer for 10 minutes or until sauce thickens. When cauliflower is done roasting, remove from oven, add it to sauce, and toss to coat. Simmer for another 2 minutes.

6. Remove from heat and serve immediately.

SPAGHETTI SQUASH SPINACH ALFREDO

Serves 6

This Spaghetti Squash Spinach Alfredo tastes like it came from your favorite Italian restaurant, but without any of the carbs. If you want to switch up the vegetables, try broccoli, asparagus, or even red bell peppers in place of the spinach.

NET CARBS
8g

Calories: 595
Fat: 58g
Sodium: 550mg
Carbohydrates: 9g
Fiber: 1g
Sugar: 5g
Sugar alcohols: 0g
Protein: 12g

INGREDIENTS

For the squash:

1 tablespoon salted grass-fed butter, melted

1 teaspoon minced garlic

1 small spaghetti squash (should be about 4½ cups cooked)

For the Alfredo sauce:

½ cup unsalted grass-fed butter

1½ teaspoons minced garlic

2 cups grass-fed heavy cream

4 ounces cream cheese, softened

¼ teaspoon sea salt

¼ teaspoon ground white pepper

⅛ teaspoon ground nutmeg

1½ cups grated Parmesan cheese

1 cup chopped spinach

1. Preheat oven to 400°F. Line a baking sheet with parchment paper and set aside.

2. Whisk together melted butter and garlic in a small bowl and spread on flesh of spaghetti squash. Arrange spaghetti squash on baking sheet, cut side down.

3. Bake for 45 minutes or until fork easily pierces squash. Remove from oven and allow to cool for 5 minutes.

4. While squash is cooling, prepare the Alfredo sauce: Melt ½ cup butter in a large skillet over medium heat. Add garlic and cook for 1 minute. Add heavy cream, cream cheese, salt, pepper, and nutmeg, and reduce heat to low.

5. Continue cooking until cream cheese melts and sauce is smooth. Slowly whisk in Parmesan cheese, stirring until sauce thickens, about 5 minutes. Stir in spinach and cook for 2 minutes or until spinach wilts.

6. Use a fork to scrape spaghetti squash strands out of the skin and add strands to sauce. Toss to coat.

7. Serve immediately.

HOMEMADE VEGGIE BURGERS

Serves 6

NET CARBS
4g

Calories: 147
Fat: 10g
Sodium: 405mg
Carbohydrates: 7g
Fiber: 3g
Sugar: 2g
Sugar alcohols: 0g
Protein: 8g

Veggie burgers are perfect for non–meat eaters on burger nights, but most traditional varieties are made with beans or potatoes as a base. This version uses finely chopped mushrooms, so it's low-carb but still hearty and satisfying.

INGREDIENTS

1 tablespoon salted grass-fed butter

½ cup finely diced sweet onion

1½ teaspoons minced garlic

8 ounces sliced baby bella mushrooms, finely chopped

1 (10-ounce) bag frozen cauliflower rice

1 teaspoon coconut aminos

1 teaspoon dried parsley

½ teaspoon sea salt

½ teaspoon ground cumin

½ teaspoon chili powder

1 cup shredded sharp Cheddar cheese

1 egg white, lightly beaten

2 tablespoons coarse almond meal

1 tablespoon chia seeds

1. Preheat oven to 400°F. Line a baking sheet with parchment paper and set aside.

2. Heat butter in a large skillet over medium heat. Add onion and cook until softened, about 5 minutes. Add garlic and cook for another minute.

3. Stir in mushrooms and cauliflower and cook for 10 minutes or until vegetables start to brown. Remove from heat.

4. Add remaining ingredients and mix well. Allow to cool for 15 minutes.

5. Divide mixture into six equal-sized balls and form each ball into a patty. Arrange in a single layer on prepared baking sheet.

6. Bake for 30 minutes or until patties turn golden brown. Remove from oven and allow to cool for 5 minutes, then serve warm.

CAULIFLOWER CASSEROLE

NET CARBS
6g

Calories: 262
Fat: 22g
Sodium: 554mg
Carbohydrates: 9g
Fiber: 3g
Sugar: 3g
Sugar alcohols: 0g
Protein: 9g

Serves 6

If you prefer a thicker casserole, replace half of the sour cream in this recipe with an equal amount of softened cream cheese. You can find fire-roasted tomatoes at most supermarkets, right next to the regular diced canned tomatoes.

INGREDIENTS

6 cups cauliflower florets

¼ cup grass-fed heavy cream

2 tablespoons salted grass-fed butter

¼ teaspoon garlic powder

¼ teaspoon onion powder

⅛ teaspoon paprika

½ teaspoon sea salt

¼ teaspoon ground black pepper

1½ cups shredded Cheddar cheese, divided

½ cup drained canned fire-roasted diced tomatoes

½ cup sour cream

2 tablespoons diced jalapeño

½ cup sliced black olives

1. Preheat oven to 350°F.

2. Bring a large pot of water to a boil and add cauliflower florets. Boil until fork-tender, about 8 minutes. Drain and transfer cauliflower to a food processor or blender.

3. Add heavy cream, butter, garlic powder, onion powder, paprika, salt, and pepper, and process until smooth. Add ½ cup cheese and stir until combined.

4. Transfer cauliflower mixture to an ungreased 9" × 9" baking pan and spread out evenly. Spread diced tomatoes on top of cauliflower and sour cream on top of tomatoes. Sprinkle with remaining cheese, jalapeño, and olives.

5. Bake for 45 minutes or until cheese is melted and casserole is bubbly. Remove from oven and allow to cool for 5 minutes, then serve warm.

PORTOBELLO MUSHROOM PIZZAS

Serves 4 (Makes 8 pizzas)

Pizza is a classic favorite, but there will probably be days when you just won't feel like putting in the effort to make a keto dough. That's when these Portobello Mushroom Pizzas are a great choice. Instead of using dough, pile all your favorite pizza toppings right into the cap of a filling portobello mushroom.

INGREDIENTS

8 large portobello mushrooms, stems removed

1 tablespoon olive oil

1 teaspoon minced garlic

¼ teaspoon sea salt

¼ teaspoon ground black pepper

1 cup Rao's Homemade Marinara Sauce

½ teaspoon dried oregano

2 cups shredded whole milk mozzarella cheese

¼ cup grated Parmesan cheese

½ cup chopped fresh basil

1. Position oven rack in center of oven. Preheat broiler on high. Line a baking sheet with parchment paper.

2. Arrange mushrooms stem side up on prepared baking sheet.

3. Combine olive oil and garlic in a small bowl and brush mixture on the insides of the mushrooms. Sprinkle with salt and pepper.

4. Broil for 5 minutes, watching carefully so mushrooms don't burn.

5. Remove from broiler.

6. Add marinara sauce and oregano to a small bowl and stir to combine. Scoop 2 tablespoons sauce into each mushroom cap.

7. Sprinkle ¼ cup mozzarella and ½ tablespoon Parmesan on top of each mushroom.

8. Broil for another 5 minutes or until cheese is melted and bubbly.

9. Remove from broiler and sprinkle with fresh basil. Allow to cool for 5 minutes, then serve warm.

SPINACH PIE

Serves 12

This Spinach Pie uses almond flour and butter to create a low-carb crust that's reminiscent of pastry dough. Although the nutmeg may seem out of place, it gives your crust a slightly nutty flavor that goes perfectly with the spinach.

NET CARBS
3g

Calories: 211
Fat: 18g
Sodium: 277mg
Carbohydrates: 6g
Fiber: 3g
Sugar: 2g
Sugar alcohols: 0g
Protein: 9g

INGREDIENTS

For the crust:

1¾ cups almond flour

½ teaspoon sea salt

¼ cup unsalted grass-fed butter, melted

1 large egg, lightly beaten

⅛ teaspoon ground nutmeg

For the filling:

1 (10-ounce) package frozen chopped spinach, thawed and drained

1 small shallot, peeled and finely chopped

¾ cup crumbled feta cheese

3 ounces cream cheese, softened

½ cup shredded whole milk mozzarella cheese

1 teaspoon minced garlic

¼ teaspoon dried oregano

3 large eggs, lightly beaten

1. Preheat oven to 350°F. Lightly grease a 9" pie plate and set aside.

2. To make the crust, combine flour and salt in a medium bowl. Add melted butter and egg and mix well. Stir in nutmeg.

3. Press mixture into the bottom of prepared pie plate. Bake for 10 minutes or until crust turns slightly golden brown.

4. To make the filling, combine filling ingredients in a large bowl and whisk to incorporate.

5. Pour filling on top of baked crust and bake for 30 minutes or until set.

6. Remove from oven and allow to cool for 5 minutes, then serve warm.

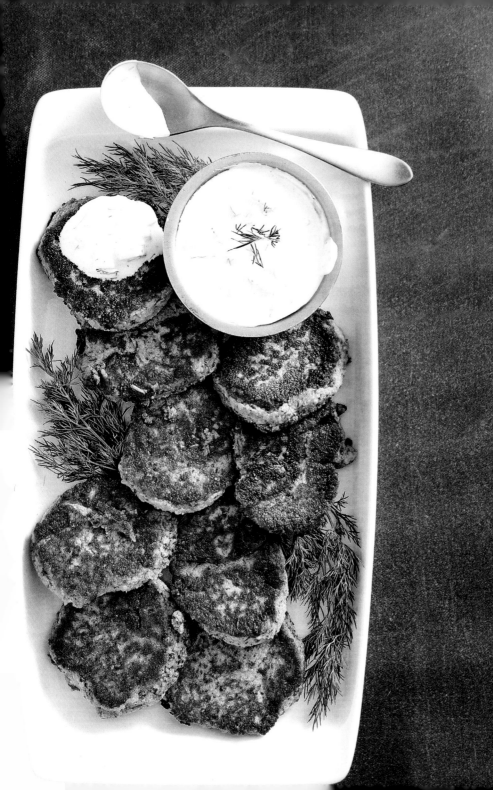

CAULIFLOWER FALAFEL WITH CUCUMBER SAUCE

NET CARBS
5g

Calories: 241
Fat: 20g
Sodium: 765mg
Carbohydrates: 12g
Fiber: 7g
Sugar: 3g
Sugar alcohols: 0g
Protein: 7g

Serves 4 (Makes 8 falafel patties)

If your cauliflower purée seems a little too soupy, use a nut milk bag or a cheesecloth to strain out some of the excess water before mixing it with the other ingredients. If you don't have an air fryer, you can carefully pan-fry the falafel in avocado oil over medium-high heat for about 10 minutes.

INGREDIENTS

For the dipping sauce:

½ cup sour cream

1 tablespoon Tessemae's Organic Mayonnaise

1 teaspoon fresh lemon juice

¼ cup finely minced cucumber

1 teaspoon dried dill

¼ teaspoon sea salt

⅛ teaspoon ground black pepper

For the falafel patties:

2 tablespoons ground flaxseed meal

¼ cup plus 2 tablespoons water

1 cup cauliflower purée (see sidebar)

½ cup coarse almond meal

1 tablespoon ground cumin

2 teaspoons ground coriander

½ teaspoon curry powder

2 teaspoons dried parsley

1 teaspoon sea salt

½ teaspoon cayenne pepper

3 tablespoons coconut flour

1 tablespoon Nature's Promise Organic Sesame Tahini

1. To make the dipping sauce, combine dipping sauce ingredients in a small bowl and whisk well. Refrigerate for 30 minutes.

2. To make the falafel, combine ground flaxseed meal and water in a small bowl and let sit for 15 minutes.

3. Preheat air fryer to 375°F.

4. Combine cauliflower purée and almond meal and mix well. Add remaining falafel ingredients, including moistened flaxseed meal, and stir until combined.

5. Form mixture into eight equal-sized patties. Spray patties with avocado oil cooking spray and arrange in a single layer in the air fryer basket (you may need to work in batches).

6. Cook for 15 minutes or until outside turns golden brown. Repeat with any remaining patties.

7. Cool for 5 minutes, then serve with dipping sauce.

MAKING CAULIFLOWER PURÉE

To make cauliflower purée, take 1 large head of cauliflower and cut it into florets. Boil them in a large pot of water for 6 minutes. Remove them from the water and bake the florets in a 325°F oven for 5 minutes to remove excess moisture. Add ¾ cup grass-fed heavy cream and process or blend until smooth.

ROSEMARY FLATBREAD

Serves 6

Similar in taste and texture to naan, this Rosemary Flatbread is delicious on its own (with some butter) or as a sandwich bread. You can even use it to make individual-sized pizzas.

NET CARBS
4g

Calories: 382
Fat: 31g
Sodium: 602mg
Carbohydrates: 7g
Fiber: 3g
Sugar: 2g
Sugar alcohols: 0g
Protein: 20g

INGREDIENTS

3 cups shredded whole milk mozzarella cheese

1 ounce cream cheese

2 large eggs, lightly beaten

1½ cups almond flour

1 tablespoon baking powder

2 tablespoons salted grass-fed butter, melted

¾ teaspoon minced garlic

1 tablespoon fresh chopped rosemary

1. Preheat oven to 375°F. Line a baking sheet with parchment paper and set aside.

2. Combine mozzarella and cream cheese in a large microwave-safe bowl and microwave on high for 60 seconds. Stir, return to microwave, and microwave on high for another 45 seconds or until cheese is melted. Stir well to combine.

3. Stir in eggs. Then add flour and baking powder and use your hands to knead ingredients together until incorporated.

4. Divide dough into six equal portions and roll each portion into a ball. Press each dough ball flat and spread out slightly to form a flatbread shape.

5. Arrange on prepared baking sheet. Bake for 8 minutes or until the top of the bread turns slightly golden brown. Remove from oven.

6. Combine butter, garlic, and rosemary in a small bowl, and brush evenly on each flatbread. Return to oven and bake for another 2 minutes.

7. Remove from oven and allow to cool for 5 minutes, then serve warm.

CHAPTER 9

SIDE DISHES

FRESH BROCCOLI SLAW

Serves 6

If you can't find a bag of broccoli slaw, you can make your own by saving your broccoli stems next time you make florets and shredding them with a cheese grater.

Calories: 30
Fat: 1g
Sodium: 280mg
Carbohydrates: 6g
Fiber: 1g
Sugar: 1g
Sugar alcohols: 3g
Protein: 1g

INGREDIENTS

⅓ cup Tessemae's Organic Mayonnaise

1 tablespoon apple cider vinegar

1 tablespoon Dijon mustard

1½ tablespoons Swerve Granular sweetener

½ teaspoon sea salt

¼ teaspoon ground black pepper

1 (12-ounce) bag broccoli slaw

1. Whisk mayonnaise, vinegar, mustard, sweetener, salt, and pepper together in a medium bowl.

2. Add broccoli slaw and toss to coat.

3. Refrigerate for 1 hour before serving.

CHEESY GARLIC BROCCOLI FLORETS

Serves 6

This side dish is easy to make and goes well with any of the main dishes in this book. You can even whip it up as a quick snack.

Calories: 121
Fat: 9g
Sodium: 138mg
Carbohydrates: 7g
Fiber: 2g
Sugar: 2g
Sugar alcohols: 0g
Protein: 5g

INGREDIENTS

1 large head broccoli, cut into bite-sized florets

½ cup water

3 tablespoons salted grass-fed butter

½ teaspoon garlic salt

½ cup shredded Cheddar cheese

1. Combine broccoli and water in a large saucepan over medium heat. Cook for 6 minutes or until broccoli is fork-tender. Drain water from saucepan and add butter.

2. Return saucepan to stovetop and reduce heat to low. Once butter is melted, toss to coat broccoli. Sprinkle garlic salt on top of broccoli and toss to coat again.

3. Stir in cheese. Continue stirring until cheese melts.

4. Remove from heat and serve immediately.

ROASTED GARLIC AND LEMON BROCCOLI

Serves 6

Roasting broccoli is an excellent way to bring out its natural sweetness. This recipe uses a lemon and garlic combination, but you can easily add some variety to the recipe by using other combinations, like Parmesan cheese and crushed red pepper flakes, or adding some hemp seeds for crunch.

Calories: 60
Fat: 4g
Sodium: 411mg
Carbohydrates: 5g
Fiber: 2g
Sugar: 1g
Sugar alcohols: 0g
Protein: 2g

INGREDIENTS

1 large head broccoli (about 1½ pounds), cut into florets

2 tablespoons unsalted grass-fed butter, melted

1 teaspoon fresh lemon juice

2 teaspoons minced garlic

1 teaspoon sea salt

½ teaspoon ground black pepper

1. Preheat oven to 400°F. Line a baking sheet with parchment paper and set aside.

2. Place broccoli in a large bowl and set aside.

3. Whisk together butter, lemon juice, and garlic in a separate small bowl. Pour over broccoli and toss to combine.

4. Spread broccoli in an even layer on prepared baking sheet. Sprinkle salt and pepper on top.

5. Bake for 20 minutes or until broccoli is fork-tender and starts to crisp.

6. Remove from oven and serve immediately.

FRIED SHAVED BRUSSELS SPROUTS

Serves 6

You can find shaved Brussels sprouts at Trader Joe's grocery stores, but if there isn't one in your area, you can grate your own Brussels sprouts using a cheese grater. Just make sure to watch your fingers!

Calories: 61
Fat: 3g
Sodium: 361mg
Carbohydrates: 7g
Fiber: 2g
Sugar: 2g
Sugar alcohols: 2g
Protein: 5g

INGREDIENTS

- 6 slices Applegate Naturals No Sugar Bacon, chopped
- 1 small sweet onion, peeled and diced
- ½ teaspoon minced garlic
- 1 (10-ounce) package Trader Joe's Shaved Brussels Sprouts
- 1 tablespoon Swerve Granular sweetener
- ½ teaspoon sea salt
- ¼ teaspoon ground black pepper

1. Heat bacon in a medium skillet over medium-high heat. Cook for 7 minutes or until browned and crispy. Transfer bacon to a paper towel–lined plate, reserving bacon grease in the skillet.

2. Reduce heat to medium and add onion to skillet. Cook for 7 minutes or until onion softens and caramelizes. Add garlic and cook for an additional minute.

3. Add shaved Brussels sprouts and stir to coat. Cook sprouts for 6 minutes or until tender and starting to brown.

4. Sprinkle sweetener, salt, and pepper on Brussels sprouts and stir to combine. Cover and cook for another 2 minutes.

5. Stir and remove from heat. Serve immediately.

JALAPEÑO POPPER MASHED CAULIFLOWER

Serves 6

This Jalapeño Popper Mashed Cauliflower gives you all the spicy, creamy taste of jalapeño poppers but without the hassle of stuffing, filling, and wrapping them. You can stir in some crispy bacon after puréeing to kick the flavor up a notch.

NET CARBS
7g

Calories: 190
Fat: 16g
Sodium: 301mg
Carbohydrates: 10g
Fiber: 3g
Sugar: 4g
Sugar alcohols: 0g
Protein: 4g

INGREDIENTS

1 large head cauliflower, cut into florets

½ cup water

¼ cup unsalted grass-fed butter

1 medium jalapeño, seeded and diced

3 green onions, trimmed and finely chopped

1 teaspoon minced garlic

4 ounces cream cheese, softened

¼ cup sour cream

½ teaspoon sea salt

¼ teaspoon ground black pepper

1. Combine cauliflower and water in a large pot over medium heat. Cover and allow cauliflower to steam until soft, about 8 minutes. Drain and transfer cauliflower to a food processor.

2. Heat butter in a small skillet over medium heat. Add jalapeño, onions, and garlic, and cook until softened, about 3 minutes.

3. Add vegetable mixture to food processor along with cream cheese, sour cream, salt, and black pepper. Pulse until smooth.

4. Serve immediately.

SPICY ROASTED CABBAGE

Serves 4

This Spicy Roasted Cabbage is the perfect low-carb side to accompany any protein dish. Try it with the Garlic and Herb–Roasted Turkey (see recipe in Chapter 5) or the Steak Tips with Gravy (see recipe in Chapter 6).

NET CARBS
2g

Calories: 76
Fat: 7g
Sodium: 359mg
Carbohydrates: 3g
Fiber: 1g
Sugar: 1g
Sugar alcohols: 0g
Protein: 2g

INGREDIENTS

- ½ large head Napa cabbage, cored and cut into 4 wedges
- 2 tablespoons Nutiva Organic Liquid Coconut Oil with Garlic
- ¼ teaspoon garlic powder
- ¼ teaspoon cayenne pepper
- ½ teaspoon sea salt
- ½ teaspoon ground black pepper

1. Preheat oven to 425°F. Line a baking sheet with parchment paper.

2. Arrange cabbage wedges on prepared baking sheet, cut side up.

3. Brush coconut oil evenly on cut edges of cabbage wedges.

4. Combine garlic powder, cayenne pepper, salt, and black pepper in a small bowl. Sprinkle mixture over cabbage. Cover cabbage loosely with foil.

5. Roast for 20 minutes, remove foil, and roast for an additional 10 minutes or until cabbage is tender.

6. Remove from oven and serve immediately.

YELLOW SQUASH CASSEROLE

NET CARBS
3g

Calories: 248
Fat: 21g
Sodium: 529mg
Carbohydrates: 4g
Fiber: 1g
Sugar: 3g
Sugar alcohols: 0g
Protein: 11g

Serves 5

Although this recipe calls for yellow squash, it's a great way to use up all of your garden zucchini in the summer too. You can use equal parts yellow squash and zucchini, or all of one or the other.

INGREDIENTS

- 4 tablespoons salted grass-fed butter, divided
- 3 cups sliced yellow squash
- ¼ cup chopped yellow onion
- 1 teaspoon minced garlic
- ½ cup shredded white Cheddar cheese
- 1 large egg, lightly beaten
- ⅓ cup grass-fed heavy cream
- ½ teaspoon sea salt
- ¼ teaspoon ground black pepper
- ½ cup crushed EPIC Oven Baked Pink Himalayan and Sea Salt Pork Rinds

1. Preheat oven to 400°F.

2. Heat 1 tablespoon butter in a large skillet over medium heat. Add squash and onion and cook until squash starts to soften, about 5 minutes. Add garlic and cook for an additional minute. Transfer to an ungreased 8" × 8" baking dish.

3. Stir cheese, egg, cream, salt, and pepper into squash. Sprinkle crushed pork rinds evenly on top. Dot pork rinds with remaining butter.

4. Bake for 25 minutes or until browned and bubbly.

5. Remove from oven and allow to cool for 5 minutes, then serve warm.

GIVE YELLOW SQUASH SOME LOVE

Keto dieters give zucchini a lot of attention, but yellow squash (also called summer squash), which is just as versatile and mild flavored, often falls by the wayside. Yellow squash may be slightly higher in net carbs—one medium yellow squash has 4.8 grams of net carbs compared to the 4 grams in a zucchini of the same size—but it's also loaded with manganese, a mineral that improves your body's ability to metabolize and process both fats and carbohydrates. If a recipe calls for zucchini and you don't have it, you can always use yellow squash in its place (or combine the two).

PAN-GLAZED MUSHROOMS

Serves 4

These Pan-Glazed Mushrooms are a tasty low-carb side dish, but they also make a great topping for steak or chicken.

INGREDIENTS

¼ cup salted grass-fed butter

1 pound sliced baby bella mushrooms

1 teaspoon minced garlic

1 tablespoon coconut aminos

¼ teaspoon ground black pepper

2 tablespoons grass-fed heavy cream

1. Melt butter in a large skillet over medium heat. Add mushrooms and cook until they start to sweat, about 5 minutes.

2. Add garlic and cook for another minute. Stir in coconut aminos and pepper and continue cooking for 4 minutes or until mixture has thickened.

3. Reduce heat to low and stir in cream. Cook for another 3 minutes or until some of the liquid evaporates.

4. Remove from heat and serve.

LEMON BUTTER AND DILL ZUCCHINI

Serves 6

You can make this recipe vegan—without sacrificing any richness or flavor—by using butter-flavored coconut oil in place of the grass-fed butter.

INGREDIENTS

¼ cup unsalted grass-fed butter

4 medium zucchini, sliced into coins

2 teaspoons dried dill

1 tablespoon fresh lemon juice

½ teaspoon sea salt

¼ teaspoon ground black pepper

1. Heat butter in a medium skillet over medium heat. Add zucchini and cook until tender, but still slightly crispy, about 4 minutes.

2. Add dill, lemon juice, salt, and pepper, and toss to coat. Cook another 2 minutes and then remove from heat.

FRIED CABBAGE

Serves 6

Cabbage is often overlooked, but it's one of the best low-carb vegetable choices. One cup of shredded cabbage contains only 2.3 grams of net carbs, but it's packed with vitamin K and vitamin C.

INGREDIENTS

6 slices Applegate Naturals No Sugar Bacon, chopped

1 medium sweet onion, peeled and finely diced

2 teaspoons minced garlic

1 large head Napa cabbage, cored and chopped

1 teaspoon sea salt

1 teaspoon ground black pepper

¼ teaspoon paprika

1. Place bacon in a large stock-pot. Cook over medium-high heat for 7 minutes or until browned and crispy. Add onion and cook for 10 minutes or until caramelized. Stir in garlic and cook for another minute.

2. Add remaining ingredients, cover, and reduce heat to low. Cook for another 20 minutes, or until cabbage is fork-tender, stirring occasionally. Remove from heat and serve immediately.

GARLIC-ROASTED MUSHROOMS

Serves 6

White mushrooms tend to have the mildest mushroom flavor, so they go well with any protein dish.

INGREDIENTS

1 pound white mushrooms, cut in half

1 teaspoon minced garlic

2 tablespoons olive oil

2 teaspoons fresh lemon juice

¼ cup chopped fresh cilantro

½ teaspoon sea salt

½ teaspoon ground black pepper

2 tablespoons unsalted grass-fed butter

1. Preheat oven to 450°F.

2. Add mushrooms, garlic, olive oil, lemon juice, cilantro, salt, and pepper to an ungreased 9" × 9" baking dish and toss to coat.

3. Spread mushrooms out and dot evenly with butter.

4. Roast 10 minutes, stir, and then roast for another 10 minutes. Remove from oven and serve.

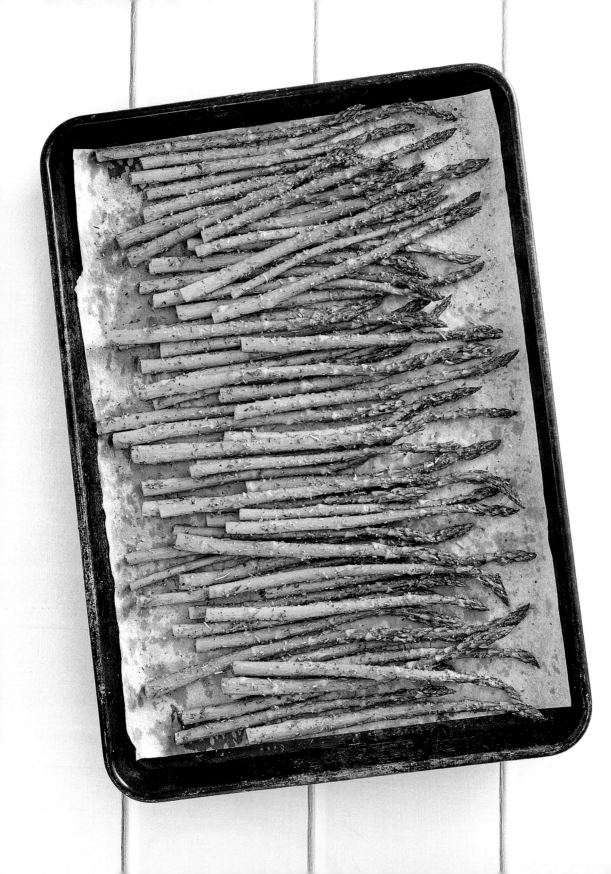

HERB-ROASTED ASPARAGUS

Serves 6

Asparagus is known for being a tough vegetable, but it's actually quite tender if you trim it right. Instead of cutting the ends off the asparagus, take each stalk in your fingers and bend it until it breaks. It will naturally break off where the tough, woody part ends and the edible part begins.

Calories: 57
Fat: 5g
Sodium: 196mg
Carbohydrates: 3g
Fiber: 2g
Sugar: 1g
Sugar alcohols: 0g
Protein: 2g

INGREDIENTS

1 pound asparagus spears, trimmed

2 tablespoons olive oil

1 teaspoon dried rosemary

1 teaspoon dried thyme

1 teaspoon dried basil

½ teaspoon sea salt

¼ teaspoon ground black pepper

1. Preheat oven to 400°F. Line a baking sheet with parchment paper and set aside.

2. Combine asparagus and olive oil in a large bowl and toss to coat. Arrange asparagus in a single layer on prepared baking sheet.

3. Sprinkle rosemary, thyme, basil, salt, and black pepper evenly over asparagus.

4. Roast for 15 minutes or until asparagus is tender and slightly brown.

5. Remove from oven and serve immediately.

CHEESY RANCH CAULIFLOWER BAKE

Serves 6

What's the best way to get out of your keto cauliflower rut? Add some ranch dressing and cheese! Tessemae's Organic Creamy Ranch Dressing is an original ranch flavor, but their other keto-friendly options, such as Habanero Ranch, Buffalo Ranch, and Everything Bagel Ranch, would work just as well here.

Calories: 340
Fat: 32g
Sodium: 718mg
Carbohydrates: 8g
Fiber: 2g
Sugar: 4g
Sugar alcohols: 0g
Protein: 7g

INGREDIENTS

5 cups cauliflower florets

½ cup water

1 teaspoon chili powder

½ teaspoon sea salt

¼ teaspoon ground black pepper

¼ cup unsalted grass-fed butter

1 cup Tessemae's Organic Creamy Ranch Dressing

1 cup shredded Cheddar cheese

1. Preheat oven to 400°F.

2. Combine cauliflower and water in a large saucepan over medium-low heat. Cover and steam for 7 minutes or until cauliflower is fork-tender.

3. Remove from heat, drain cauliflower, and return it to saucepan. Add chili powder, salt, pepper, and butter to saucepan, and stir until butter is melted and cauliflower is evenly coated.

4. Transfer cauliflower to an ungreased 8" × 8" baking dish and pour ranch dressing on top. Toss to coat.

5. Sprinkle cheese on top of cauliflower and bake for 15 minutes or until cheese is melted and cauliflower is hot and bubbly.

6. Remove from oven and allow to cool for 5 minutes, then serve warm.

SPICY CHILI KALE CHIPS

Serves 4

NET CARBS
1g

Calories: 42
Fat: 4g
Sodium: 626mg
Carbohydrates: 2g
Fiber: 1g
Sugar: 0g
Sugar alcohols: 0g
Protein: 1g

When preparing kale, remove the tough central stalk (called the rib) and reserve the leaf pieces only. Cut them into bite-sized pieces and then proceed with recipe.

INGREDIENTS

4 cups chopped kale

1 tablespoon olive oil

2 teaspoons chili powder

1 teaspoon sea salt

⅛ teaspoon cayenne pepper

1. Preheat oven to 400°F. Line a baking sheet with parchment paper and set aside.

2. Place kale in a large bowl and drizzle olive oil on top. Toss to coat.

3. Arrange kale in a single layer on prepared baking sheet. Sprinkle chili powder, salt, and cayenne pepper on kale.

4. Roast for 5 minutes, stir kale, and rearrange in a single layer. Roast for another 5 minutes or until kale is browned and crispy. Remove from oven and serve.

ROASTED OKRA

Serves 4

NET CARBS
3g

Calories: 78
Fat: 6g
Sodium: 543mg
Carbohydrates: 6g
Fiber: 3g
Sugar: 3g
Sugar alcohols: 0g
Protein: 2g

Okra contains only 1.9 grams of net carbs per ½-cup serving, but it's packed with antioxidants and vitamins.

INGREDIENTS

1 pound okra, sliced in half lengthwise

2 tablespoons salted grass-fed butter, melted

1 teaspoon garlic salt

1 teaspoon ground black pepper

¼ teaspoon ground cumin

¼ teaspoon ground coriander

1. Preheat oven to 425°F. Line a baking sheet with parchment paper and set aside.

2. Combine okra and butter and in a large bowl and toss to coat. Arrange okra in a single layer on prepared baking sheet.

3. Sprinkle garlic salt, pepper, cumin, and coriander evenly on top of okra.

4. Bake for 15 minutes or until fork-tender.

5. Remove from oven and serve immediately.

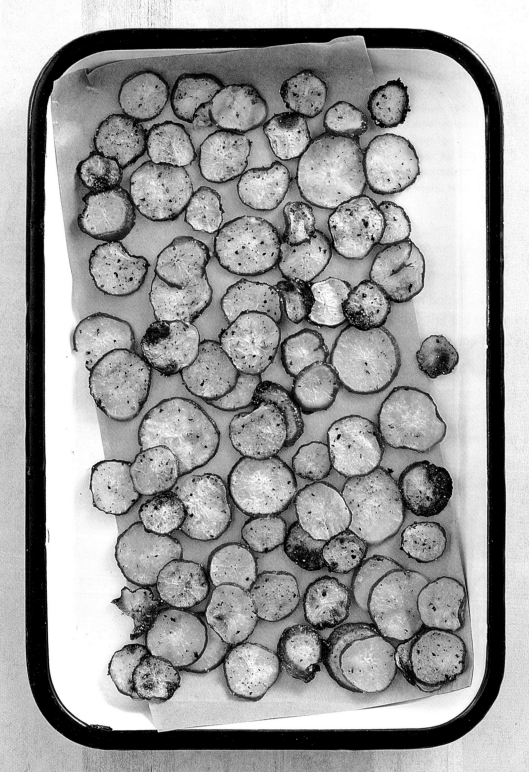

Salt and Vinegar Radish Chips

SALT AND VINEGAR RADISH CHIPS

Serves 6

Radishes are little, but they pack a big crunch.

NET CARBS
2g

Calories: 53
Fat: 5g
Sodium: 224mg
Carbohydrates: 3g
Fiber: 1g
Sugar: 1g
Sugar alcohols: 0g
Protein: 1g

INGREDIENTS

2 tablespoons olive oil

1 tablespoon apple cider vinegar

1 pound fresh radishes, sliced thinly, using a mandoline if possible

½ teaspoon sea salt

½ teaspoon ground black pepper

1. Preheat oven to 400°F. Line two baking sheets with parchment paper and set aside.

2. Whisk together olive oil and vinegar in a medium mixing bowl. Add radishes and toss to coat.

3. Arrange radish slices in a single layer on prepared baking sheets. Sprinkle salt and pepper over slices.

4. Bake 15 minutes. Remove from oven and serve immediately.

GARLIC BUTTER–ROASTED CAULIFLOWER

Serves 6

You'll be surprised at how rich and delicious this Garlic Butter–Roasted Cauliflower is with only five simple ingredients.

NET CARBS
4g

Calories: 87
Fat: 6g
Sodium: 430mg
Carbohydrates: 7g
Fiber: 3g
Sugar: 3g
Sugar alcohols: 0g
Protein: 3g

INGREDIENTS

3 tablespoons unsalted grass-fed butter, melted

1 teaspoon minced garlic

1 large head cauliflower, cut into florets

1 teaspoon sea salt

½ teaspoon ground black pepper

1. Preheat oven to 425°F. Line a baking sheet with parchment paper and set aside.

2. Whisk butter and garlic together in a large bowl. Add cauliflower and toss to coat evenly.

3. Spread cauliflower out on prepared baking sheet and sprinkle with salt and pepper.

4. Roast for 20 minutes, flip cauliflower over, and roast for another 20 minutes. Remove from oven and serve.

BREADLESS BROCCOLI GRATIN

Serves 8

This Breadless Broccoli Gratin is perfectly cheesy and delicious as is, but if you want to add some crunch, make a low-carb "breaded" topping by adding some crushed pork rinds and a few pats of butter on top before baking.

INGREDIENTS

8 cups broccoli florets

½ cup water

2 small shallots, peeled and chopped

¼ cup unsalted grass-fed butter

½ teaspoon xanthan gum

1 cup grass-fed heavy cream

1 teaspoon sea salt

½ teaspoon ground black pepper

¼ teaspoon crushed red pepper flakes

½ teaspoon ground nutmeg

3 cups shredded white Cheddar cheese

2 large eggs, lightly beaten

1. Preheat oven to 350°F.

2. Combine broccoli and water in a large stockpot over medium-high heat. Cook for 4 minutes or until broccoli turns bright green and slightly tender.

3. Drain broccoli and transfer to an ungreased 9" × 13" baking dish and mix in shallots. Set aside.

4. Melt butter in a small saucepan over medium heat. Whisk in xanthan gum and cook until mixture bubbles, about 2 minutes.

5. Slowly whisk in cream and bring to a low boil. Remove from heat and stir in salt, black pepper, red pepper flakes, and nutmeg. Add cheese a little at a time, stirring to incorporate after each addition.

6. Once all cheese is melted and smooth, allow to cool for 3 minutes, then add eggs to mixture and stir to incorporate.

7. Pour cheese mixture over broccoli and stir to combine. Spread broccoli out evenly in baking dish and bake for 30 minutes or until mixture is hot and bubbly.

8. Remove from oven and allow to cool for 5 minutes, then serve warm.

PARMESAN RAINBOW CHARD

NET CARBS

6g

Calories: **185**
Fat: **14g**
Sodium: **553mg**
Carbohydrates: **8g**
Fiber: **2g**
Sugar: **4g**
Sugar alcohols: **0g**
Protein: **5g**

Serves 4

Rainbow chard adds some color and character to this finished dish, but if you can't find it, you can use regular Swiss chard in its place for equally delicious results. Either way, you'll get a hefty dose of potassium, magnesium, and calcium, minerals that are essential for a healthy heart.

INGREDIENTS

3 tablespoons salted grass-fed butter

¼ cup minced yellow onion

2 teaspoons minced garlic

6 cups finely chopped rainbow chard

½ cup FitVine Pinot Grigio

2 teaspoons fresh lemon juice

2 tablespoons shredded Parmesan cheese

½ teaspoon sea salt

3 tablespoons grass-fed heavy cream

1. Heat butter in a large skillet over medium heat. Add onion and cook for 3 minutes. Stir in garlic and cook for an additional minute.

2. Add chard and wine to the skillet, stir, and cover. Simmer for 7 minutes or until stems are fork-tender.

3. Stir in lemon juice, cheese, and salt. Add cream and simmer for another 2 minutes.

4. Remove from heat and serve.

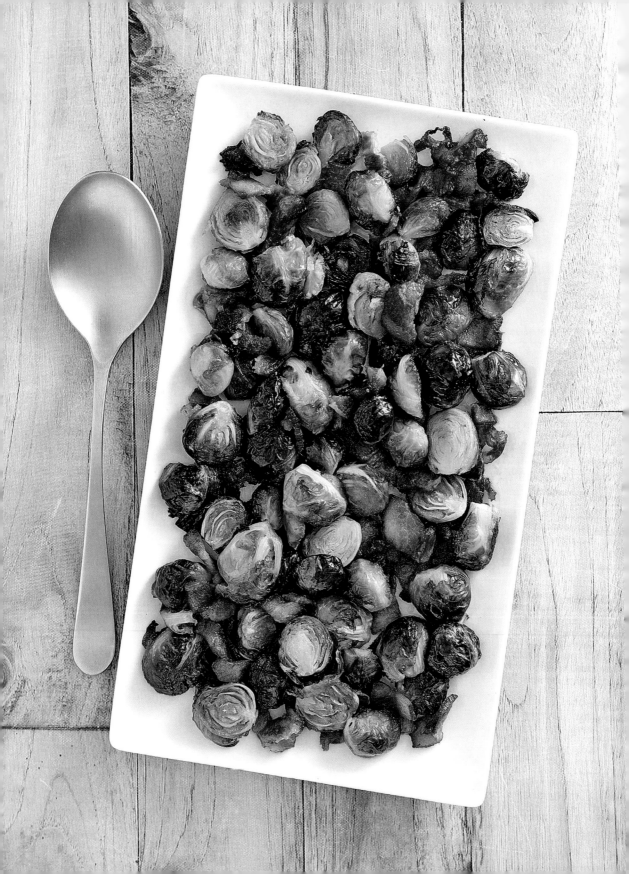

MAPLE-ROASTED BRUSSELS SPROUTS

Serves 6

If you thought bacon and Brussels sprouts were a good combo, wait until you try them with bacon and this keto-friendly maple syrup. Serve these Maple-Roasted Brussels Sprouts alongside the Roasted Leg of Lamb (see recipe in Chapter 6) for a real treat.

NET CARBS

4g

Calories: 140
Fat: 10g
Sodium: 320mg
Carbohydrates: 14g
Fiber: 10g
Sugar: 2g
Sugar alcohols: 0g
Protein: 5g

INGREDIENTS

¼ cup unsalted grass-fed butter, melted

3 tablespoons ChocZero Maple Syrup

1 pound Brussels sprouts, trimmed and halved

4 slices Applegate Naturals No Sugar Bacon, roughly chopped

½ teaspoon sea salt

1. Preheat oven to 400°F. Line a baking sheet with parchment paper and set aside.

2. Whisk together butter and maple syrup in a large bowl. Add Brussels sprouts and chopped bacon to bowl and toss to coat.

3. Spread evenly in a single layer on prepared baking sheet. Sprinkle with salt.

4. Bake for 20 minutes or until Brussels sprouts are tender and bacon is crisp.

5. Remove from oven and serve immediately.

CHAPTER 10

FAT BOMBS

CINNAMON ROLL FAT BOMBS

Serves 12

Who says you can't have buns of steel *and* buns of cinnamon? These fat bombs give you all the flavor of a cinnamon roll without throwing you out of ketosis and getting in the way of your fitness goals.

NET CARBS
2g

Calories: 102
Fat: 10g
Sodium: 60mg
Carbohydrates: 8g
Fiber: 0g
Sugar: 1g
Sugar alcohols: 6g
Protein: 2g

INGREDIENTS

4 ounces cream cheese, softened

4 tablespoons salted grass-fed butter, softened

¼ cup creamy no-sugar-added unsalted sunflower seed butter

¼ cup plus 2 tablespoons Swerve Granular sweetener, divided

1½ teaspoons ground cinnamon, divided

1 teaspoon vanilla extract

1. Line a baking sheet with parchment paper and set aside.

2. Combine cream cheese and grass-fed butter in a medium bowl and beat with a handheld electric mixer on medium until incorporated and fluffy. Beat in sunflower seed butter, ¼ cup sweetener, 1 teaspoon cinnamon, and vanilla until smooth.

3. Refrigerate for 2 hours. Divide mixture into twelve equal-sized portions and roll each portion into a ball.

4. Combine remaining sweetener and remaining cinnamon in a small bowl. Roll each fat bomb in cinnamon mixture until coated and arrange on prepared baking sheet.

5. Transfer to refrigerator and chill until set, about 2 hours. Store in an airtight container in the refrigerator for up to 2 weeks or in the freezer for up to 6 months.

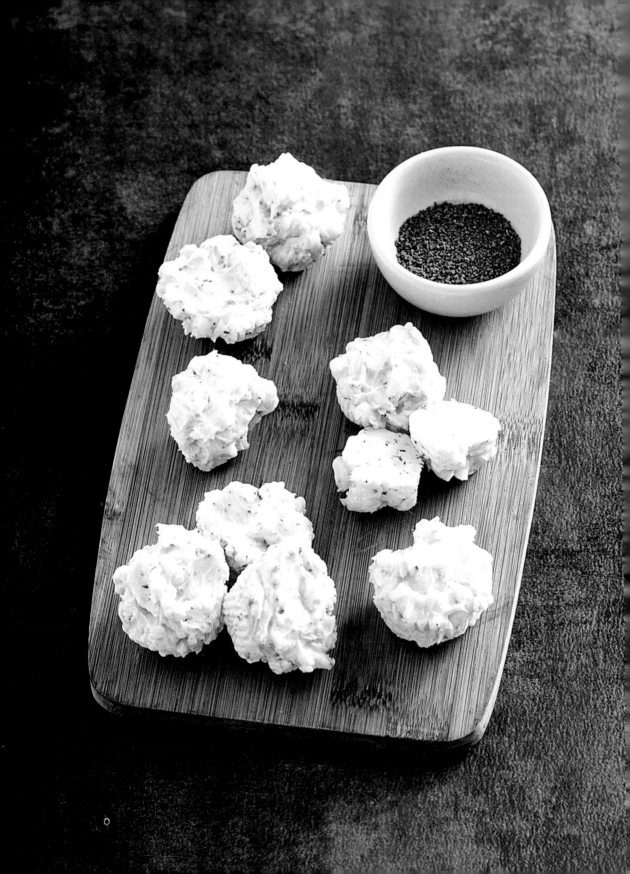

MATCHA GREEN TEA FAT BOMBS

Serves 12

When it comes to matcha, a little goes a long way, so stick to the amount in the ingredient list. It may not seem like a lot, but the flavor will really come through, especially if you use a high-quality matcha.

NET CARBS
2g

Calories: 133
Fat: 13g
Sodium: 59mg
Carbohydrates: 8g
Fiber: 2g
Sugar: 1g
Sugar alcohols: 4g
Protein: 1g

INGREDIENTS

½ cup Wildly Organic Coconut Butter, softened

8 ounces cream cheese, softened

1 teaspoon vanilla extract

½ teaspoon matcha green tea powder

⅓ cup Swerve Confectioners sweetener

1. Line twelve cups of a mini muffin pan with paper liners, or use a mini silicone muffin pan without liners. Set aside.

2. Combine all ingredients in a large bowl and beat with a handheld electric mixer on medium speed until smooth.

3. Pour equal amounts of mixture into twelve cups of the prepared muffin pan.

4. Transfer to refrigerator and chill until set, about 2 hours. Store in an airtight container in the refrigerator for up to 2 weeks or in the freezer for up to 6 months.

HEALTH BENEFITS OF MATCHA

Matcha is a powdered green tea that brings a bold taste and impressive health benefits. All green tea contains the catechin EGCG, but matcha has at least three times more than that of other green teas. EGCG can help reduce inflammation, promote a healthy weight, and help prevent heart disease and brain problems. Matcha has also been shown to protect the liver and improve brain function.

LEMON CHEESECAKE FAT BOMBS

Serves 12

The coconut butter in these fat bombs helps keep them firm, but if you don't have any, you can replace it with Perfect Keto Nut Butter or any other low-carb nut butter. Just make sure to keep an eye on your net carbs!

NET CARBS
2g

Calories: 132
Fat: 13g
Sodium: 59mg
Carbohydrates: 8g
Fiber: 2g
Sugar: 1g
Sugar alcohols: 4g
Protein: 1g

INGREDIENTS

½ cup Wildly Organic Coconut Butter, softened

8 ounces cream cheese, softened

1 teaspoon fresh lemon juice

½ teaspoon lemon zest

⅓ cup Swerve Confectioners sweetener

1. Line twelve cups of a mini muffin pan with paper liners, or use a mini silicone muffin pan without liners. Set aside.

2. Combine all ingredients in a medium bowl and beat with a handheld electric mixer on medium speed until smooth.

3. Pour equal amounts of mixture into twelve cups of the prepared muffin pan.

4. Transfer to refrigerator and chill until set, about 2 hours. Store in an airtight container in the refrigerator for up to 2 weeks or in the freezer for up to 6 months.

EVERYTHING BAGEL BOMBS

Serves 12

These Everything Bagel Bombs give you all the taste of a toasted everything bagel with cream cheese, but without any of the carbs. They're perfect alongside your morning cup of coffee.

NET CARBS

1g

Calories: 50
Fat: 5g
Sodium: 46mg
Carbohydrates: 1g
Fiber: 0g
Sugar: 0g
Sugar alcohols: 0g
Protein: 1g

INGREDIENTS

5 ounces cream cheese, softened

1 tablespoon salted grass-fed butter, softened

1 tablespoon dried chives

2 tablespoons Trader Joe's Everything But the Bagel Sesame Seasoning Blend

1. Line a baking sheet with parchment paper and set aside.

2. Combine cream cheese and butter in a medium bowl and beat with a handheld electric mixer on medium speed until incorporated and fluffy. Stir in chives.

3. Chill in the refrigerator for 1 hour or until mixture firms slightly. Use wet hands to form mixture into twelve balls. Roll each ball in bagel seasoning to lightly coat.

4. Arrange balls on prepared baking sheet and refrigerate for 2 hours. Store in an airtight container in the refrigerator for up to 2 weeks.

CHOCOLATE MACADAMIA FAT BOMBS

NET CARBS
1g

Serves 12

Macadamia nuts are the ideal keto diet choice. They're the highest-fat nut—coming in at 21 grams of fat per 1-ounce serving—and one of the lowest in carbs. A single serving of macadamia nuts has only 1.5 grams of net carbs.

Calories: 146
Fat: 15g
Sodium: 25mg
Carbohydrates: 3g
Fiber: 2g
Sugar: 0g
Sugar alcohols: 0g
Protein: 2g

INGREDIENTS

½ cup macadamia nut butter

¼ cup raw cacao powder

¼ cup Nutiva Organic Coconut Oil with Buttery Flavor, melted

8 drops liquid stevia

⅛ teaspoon sea salt

¼ cup crushed macadamia nuts

1. Line twelve cups of a mini muffin pan with paper liners, or use a mini silicone muffin pan without liners. Set aside.

2. Combine nut butter, cacao powder, coconut oil, stevia, and salt in a food processor and process until smooth.

3. Transfer to a medium bowl and stir in macadamia nuts.

4. Pour equal amounts of mixture into twelve cups of the prepared muffin pan.

5. Transfer to refrigerator and chill until set, about 2 hours. Store in an airtight container in the refrigerator for up to 2 weeks or in the freezer for up to 6 months.

THE MANY BENEFITS OF MACADAMIAS

Macadamia nuts aren't only low in net carbs and high in healthy fats; they have lots of other health benefits too. Studies show that macadamia nuts may help reduce your risk of heart disease, metabolic syndrome, and certain types of cancers. Macadamia nuts are also connected to good gut and brain health and can help aid in weight loss.

PEPPERMINT MOCHA FAT BOMBS

Serves 12

If you don't have coffee extract, you can use a small amount of strongly brewed coffee instead. It won't change the carbohydrate count, but you may have to add a little extra cream cheese to get the right consistency.

INGREDIENTS

¼ cup salted grass-fed butter, softened

¼ cup Nutiva Organic Coconut Oil with Buttery Flavor, softened

2 ounces cream cheese, softened

2 tablespoons raw cacao powder

½ teaspoon coffee extract

¼ teaspoon peppermint extract

3 tablespoons Swerve Confectioners sweetener

1. Line twelve cups of a mini muffin pan with paper liners, or use a mini silicone muffin pan without liners. Set aside.

2. Combine butter, coconut oil, and cream cheese in a medium bowl and beat with a handheld electric mixer on medium speed until smooth. Add cacao powder, coffee extract, peppermint extract, and sweetener, and beat until smooth.

3. Pour equal amounts of mixture into twelve cups of the prepared muffin pan.

4. Transfer to refrigerator and chill until set, about 2 hours. Store in an airtight container in the refrigerator for up to 2 weeks or in the freezer for up to 6 months.

PEANUT BUTTER CHEESECAKE FAT BOMBS

NET CARBS
3g

Calories: 129
Fat: 12g
Sodium: 43mg
Carbohydrates: 7g
Fiber: 1g
Sugar: 2g
Sugar alcohols: 3g
Protein: 4g

Serves 12

If peanut butter doesn't fit into your macros for the day, you can use Perfect Keto Nut Butter. The Chocolate Hazelnut flavor is a blend of macadamia nuts, other nuts, and coconut. It has only 2 grams of net carbs per 2-tablespoon serving (many peanut butters have 4 grams) and 16 grams of healthy fats, including MCTs.

INGREDIENTS

⅔ cup no-sugar-added creamy peanut butter

⅔ cup cream cheese, softened

3 tablespoons Swerve Granular sweetener

1. Line a baking sheet with parchment paper and set aside.

2. Combine peanut butter and cream cheese in a medium bowl and beat with a handheld electric mixer on medium speed until smooth. Beat in sweetener until incorporated.

3. Divide mixture into twelve equal-sized portions and roll into balls. Arrange balls on prepared baking sheet.

4. Transfer to refrigerator and chill until set, about 2 hours. Store in an airtight container in the refrigerator for up to 2 weeks or in the freezer for up to 6 months.

CHOCOLATE-COVERED ESPRESSO FAT BOMBS

Serves 12

The chocolate stevia adds a little extra chocolate flavor to these Chocolate-Covered Espresso Fat Bombs, but if you don't have any, use any liquid stevia that you have.

INGREDIENTS

⅓ cup almond butter

⅓ cup coconut oil

1 tablespoon NOW Sports Chocolate Mocha MCT Oil

3 tablespoons raw cacao powder

2 tablespoons Anthony's Espresso Baking Powder

8 drops SweetLeaf Sweet Drops Chocolate Flavored Stevia Sweetener

½ teaspoon vanilla extract

⅛ teaspoon sea salt

1. Line twelve cups of a mini muffin pan with paper liners, or use a mini silicone muffin pan without liners. Set aside.

2. Combine all ingredients in a small saucepan and stir over low heat until melted and smooth, about 5 minutes.

3. Pour equal amounts of mixture into twelve cups of the prepared muffin pan.

4. Transfer to refrigerator and chill until set, about 2 hours. Store in an airtight container in the refrigerator for up to 2 weeks or in the freezer for up to 6 months.

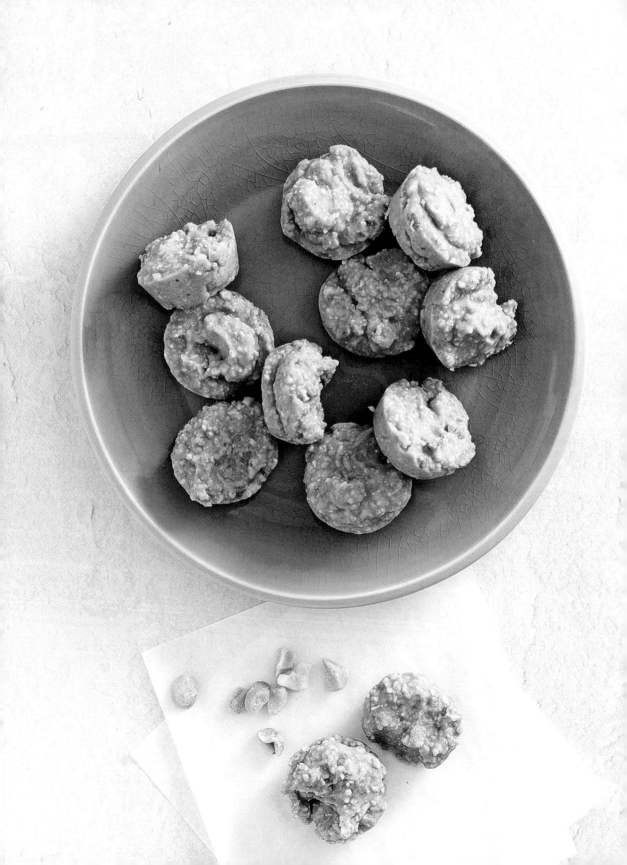

GOLDEN MILK FAT BOMBS

NET CARBS
1g

Serves 12

If you don't have California Gold Dust Superspice Mix, you can use a blend of ground turmeric, ground cinnamon, ground ginger, and ground black pepper in its place. The combination of spices adds an earthy, warming flavor that also helps combat chronic inflammation.

Calories: 171
Fat: 18g
Sodium: 1mg
Carbohydrates: 2g
Fiber: 1g
Sugar: 1g
Sugar alcohols: 0g
Protein: 1g

INGREDIENTS

1 cup raw macadamia nuts

½ cup Nutiva Organic Coconut Oil with Buttery Flavor

1 teaspoon vanilla extract

1 tablespoon Perfect Keto Vanilla MCT Oil Powder

12 drops liquid stevia

2 teaspoons California Gold Dust Superspice Mix

1. Line twelve cups of a mini muffin pan with paper liners, or use a mini silicone muffin pan without liners. Set aside.

2. Place macadamia nuts in a food processor and pulse until smooth.

3. Add coconut oil and pulse until smooth.

4. Add remaining ingredients and process until smooth.

5. Pour equal amounts of mixture into each cup of prepared muffin pan. Freeze for 2 hours.

6. Store in an airtight container in the refrigerator for up to 2 weeks or the freezer for up to 3 months.

THE PIPERINE IN BLACK PEPPER

Curcumin, which is the compound that gives turmeric all its health benefits, must be combined with black pepper in order for the body to absorb it. This is because black pepper contains a compound called piperine, which increases curcumin absorption by 2,000 percent. When making anything with turmeric, always make sure to add a little bit of black pepper, or your body won't be able to use it effectively.

PUMPKIN SPICE FAT BOMBS

Serves 12

Make sure you're getting pumpkin purée, and not pumpkin pie filling, for these fat bombs. Pumpkin purée is pure pumpkin, but pumpkin pie *filling* contains sugar and other undesirable ingredients. Although pumpkin is generally considered a high-carb vegetable, the small amount in these fat bombs won't add too many carbs.

NET CARBS
2g

Calories: 136
Fat: 14g
Sodium: 61mg
Carbohydrates: 8g
Fiber: 0g
Sugar: 1g
Sugar alcohols: 6g
Protein: 1g

INGREDIENTS

8 ounces cream cheese, softened

½ cup unsalted grass-fed butter, softened

¼ cup pumpkin purée

¼ cup plus 2 tablespoons Swerve Granular sweetener

1 teaspoon pumpkin pie spice

1. Line a baking sheet with parchment paper and set aside.

2. Combine all ingredients in a medium bowl and beat with a handheld electric mixer on medium speed until smooth.

3. Refrigerate mixture for 30 minutes to firm up.

4. Divide mixture into twelve equal-sized portions and roll into balls. Arrange balls on prepared baking sheet.

5. Transfer to refrigerator and chill until set, about 2 hours. Store in an airtight container in the refrigerator for up to 2 weeks or in the freezer for up to 6 months.

SEA SALT AND PEANUT BUTTER FAT BOMBS

Serves 12

NET CARBS
2g

Flaked sea salt typically has a stronger, saltier taste than other forms of sea salt, so measure your amount carefully.

Calories: 176
Fat: 17g
Sodium: 148mg
Carbohydrates: 3g
Fiber: 1g
Sugar: 1g
Sugar alcohols: 0g
Protein: 4g

INGREDIENTS

½ cup Nutiva Organic Coconut Oil with Buttery Flavor

¾ cup no-sugar-added creamy peanut butter

1 teaspoon vanilla extract

5 drops liquid stevia

¾ teaspoon sea salt flakes

1. Line twelve cups of a mini muffin pan with paper liners, or use a mini silicone muffin pan without liners. Set aside.

2. Combine coconut oil and peanut butter in a small saucepan over low heat. Stir until melted and combined, about 5 minutes. Stir in vanilla and stevia.

3. Pour equal amounts of mixture into twelve cups of the prepared muffin pan.

4. Sprinkle salt evenly on top of each fat bomb.

5. Transfer to refrigerator and chill until set, about 2 hours. Store in an airtight container in the refrigerator for up to 2 weeks or in the freezer for up to 6 months.

LEMON MACADAMIA FAT BOMBS

Serves 12

The macadamia nut butter adds a heap of healthy monoun-saturated fats to these Lemon Macadamia Fat Bombs. If you don't have any, you can make your own by puréeing some macadamia nuts with a little bit of macadamia nut oil until a butter forms.

NET CARBS
1g

Calories: 138
Fat: 15g
Sodium: 0mg
Carbohydrates: 2g
Fiber: 1g
Sugar: 0g
Sugar alcohols: 0g
Protein: 1g

INGREDIENTS

½ cup macadamia nut butter

¼ cup Nutiva Organic Coconut Oil with Buttery Flavor, melted

½ teaspoon lemon extract

¼ teaspoon lemon zest

8 drops liquid stevia

¼ cup crushed macadamia nuts

1. Line twelve cups of a mini muffin pan with paper liners, or use a mini silicone muffin pan without liners. Set aside.

2. Combine macadamia nut butter, coconut oil, lemon extract, lemon zest, and stevia in a food processor and process until smooth.

3. Transfer to a medium bowl and stir in macadamia nuts.

4. Pour equal amounts of mixture into twelve cups of the prepared muffin pan.

5. Transfer to refrigerator and chill until set, about 2 hours. Store in an airtight container in the refrigerator for up to 2 weeks or in the freezer for up to 6 months.

PIZZA FAT BOMBS

Serves 12

There's almost nothing better than little pizza bites that you can easily take on the go. These fat bombs combine all the delicious flavors of pepperoni pizza, but with a carb count that's appropriate for a keto diet. Store them in the refrigerator so that they keep their shape.

NET CARBS
2g

Calories: 112
Fat: 10g
Sodium: 244mg
Carbohydrates: 2g
Fiber: 0g
Sugar: 1g
Sugar alcohols: 0g
Protein: 3g

INGREDIENTS

8 ounces cream cheese, softened

½ cup chopped pepperoni

½ cup chopped black olives

¼ cup chopped fresh basil

¼ cup shredded Parmesan cheese

¼ cup no-sugar-added pizza sauce

1. Line a baking sheet with parchment paper and set aside.

2. Combine all ingredients in a medium bowl and beat with a handheld electric mixer on low speed until fully incorporated.

3. Refrigerate mixture 30 minutes.

4. Divide into twelve equal portions. Form each portion into a ball and arrange on prepared baking sheet.

5. Chill in the refrigerator for 2 hours. Store in an airtight container in the refrigerator for up to 1 week.

OLEIC ACID IN OLIVES

Around 74 percent of the fat in olives is oleic acid, a monounsaturated fat that's credited with many of the health benefits of olive oil. Oleic acid has been linked to decreased chronic inflammation, a reduced risk of heart disease, and cancer prevention. In addition to their high fat content, olives are also low in carbohydrates, which comprises only about 4 to 6 percent of their total volume. Of these carbohydrates, 52 to 86 percent comes from fiber, making the net carbohydrate count negligible. Olives make a great addition to savory fat bombs, salads, cheese bakes, and burrito bowls.

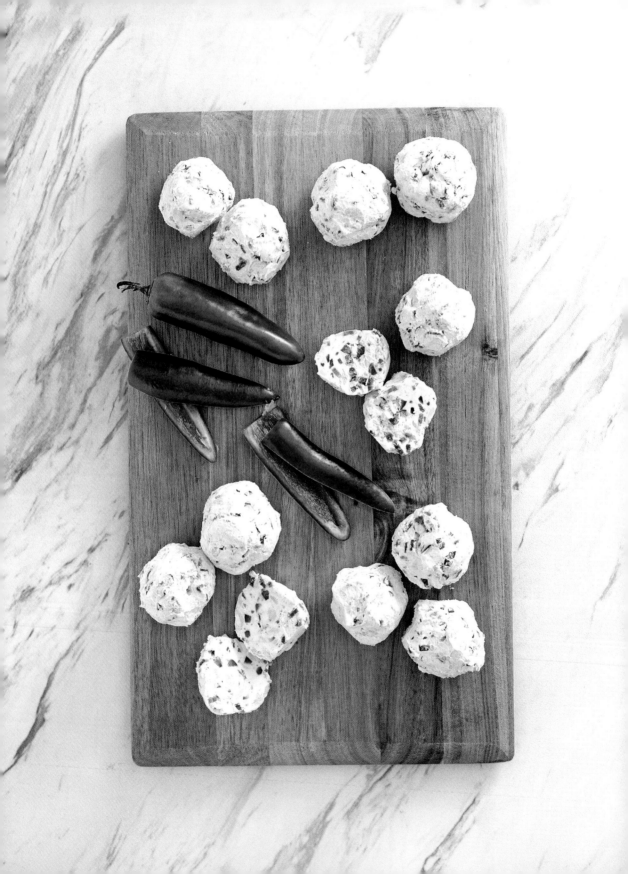

JALAPEÑO POPPER FAT BOMBS

Serves 12

You can store these Jalapeño Popper Fat Bombs in the freezer up to 3 months, so if you want to save some time down the road, double the recipe and freeze them. Thaw what you need as you go.

NET CARBS
1g

Calories: 155
Fat: 15g
Sodium: 154mg
Carbohydrates: 1g
Fiber: 0g
Sugar: 1g
Sugar alcohols: 0g
Protein: 4g

INGREDIENTS

6 ounces cream cheese, softened

½ cup unsalted grass-fed butter, softened

6 slices Applegate Naturals No Sugar Bacon, cooked and chopped

½ cup shredded Cheddar cheese

2 small jalapeños, seeded and minced

1. Line a baking sheet with parchment paper and set aside.

2. Combine cream cheese and butter in a food processor and process until smooth.

3. Add remaining ingredients and stir until incorporated.

4. Refrigerate until mixture firms up, about 1 hour.

5. Divide into twelve equal portions and roll each portion into a ball. Arrange balls on prepared baking sheet. Chill in the freezer until set, about 2 hours.

6. Store in an airtight container in the refrigerator for up to 2 weeks or in the freezer for up to 3 months.

BIRTHDAY CAKE FAT BOMBS

Serves 12

Good Dee's Sugar-Free Sprinkles are sweetened with erythritol and colored with natural-color extracts, like beet root powder and carotene powder. You may have to buy them online since they're hard to find in stores, but the extra effort is worth it!

INGREDIENTS

4 ounces cream cheese, softened

4 tablespoons unsalted grass-fed butter, softened

2 tablespoons unsweetened cashew butter

½ teaspoon almond extract

2 tablespoons almond flour

2 tablespoons Swerve Granular sweetener

2 tablespoons Good Dee's Sugar-Free Sprinkles

1. Line a baking sheet with parchment paper and set aside.

2. Combine all ingredients except sprinkles in a medium bowl and beat with a handheld electric mixer on medium speed until combined.

3. Stir in sprinkles.

4. Divide mixture into twelve equal-sized portions and roll into balls. Arrange balls on prepared baking sheet.

5. Transfer to refrigerator and chill until set, about 2 hours. Store in an airtight container in the refrigerator for up to 2 weeks or in the freezer for up to 6 months.

CHEDDAR RANCH FAT BOMBS

Serves 12

These Cheddar Ranch Fat Bombs are the perfect solution to satisfy your savory cravings. They combine the flavors of ranch with Cheddar cheese and are coated in macadamia nuts, which are loaded with monounsaturated fats, which keep your heart healthy.

NET CARBS

2g

Calories: 89
Fat: 9g
Sodium: 100mg
Carbohydrates: 2g
Fiber: 0g
Sugar: 1g
Sugar alcohols: 0g
Protein: 2g

INGREDIENTS

6 ounces cream cheese, softened

1 teaspoon garlic powder

½ teaspoon dried dill

½ teaspoon dried parsley

⅛ teaspoon sea salt

½ cup shredded Cheddar cheese

¼ cup crushed macadamia nuts

1. Line a baking sheet with parchment paper and set aside.

2. Combine cream cheese, garlic powder, dill, parsley, and salt in a medium bowl and beat with a handheld electric mixer at medium speed until smooth. Beat in Cheddar cheese.

3. Refrigerate for 1 hour or until cream hardens slightly.

4. Divide mixture into twelve equal-sized portions and roll into balls. Roll each ball in crushed macadamia nuts to coat. Arrange balls on prepared baking sheet.

5. Transfer to refrigerator and chill until set, about 2 hours. Store in an airtight container in the refrigerator for up to 2 weeks or in the freezer for up to 3 months.

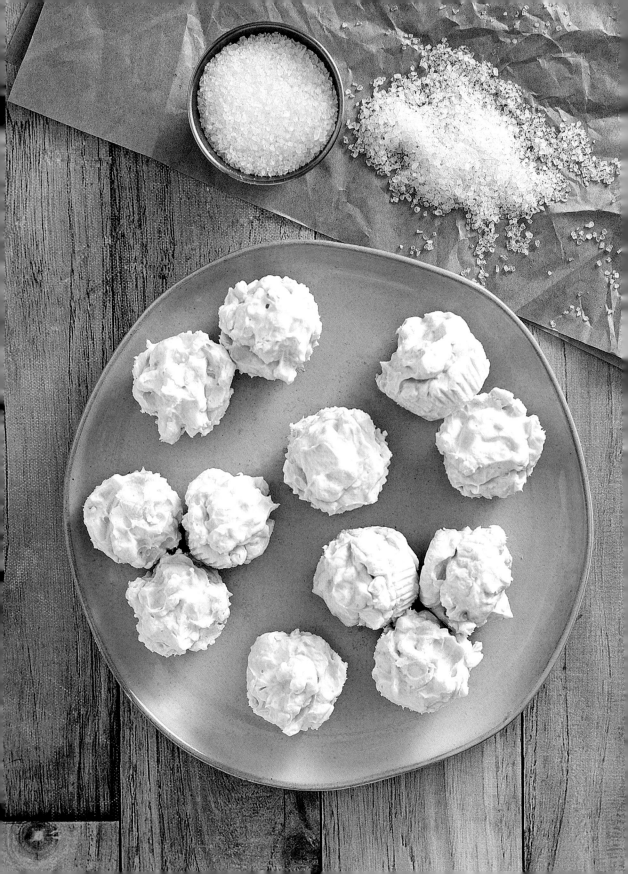

SALTED CARAMEL FAT BOMBS

Serves 12

If you don't have caramel-flavored stevia, you can use some ChocZero Caramel Syrup for these fat bombs instead. You'll probably need closer to a teaspoon, though, so if you use it, reduce the amount of cream accordingly to ensure the right consistency.

NET CARBS
1g

Calories: 118
Fat: 12g
Sodium: 174mg
Carbohydrates: 2g
Fiber: 0g
Sugar: 1g
Sugar alcohols: 1g
Protein: 1g

INGREDIENTS

8 ounces cream cheese, softened

2 tablespoons salted grass-fed butter, softened

½ cup grass-fed heavy cream

1 tablespoon Swerve Granular sweetener

½ teaspoon vanilla extract

6 drops SweetLeaf Sweet Drops Caramel Flavored Stevia Sweetener

½ teaspoon sea salt flakes

1. Line twelve cups of a mini muffin pan with paper liners, or use a mini silicone muffin pan without liners. Set aside.

2. Combine cream cheese and butter in a medium bowl and beat with a handheld electric mixer on medium speed until smooth. Beat in heavy cream, granular sweetener, vanilla, and stevia.

3. Pour equal amounts of mixture into twelve cups of the prepared muffin pan. Sprinkle salt evenly on top of each fat bomb.

4. Transfer to refrigerator and chill until set, about 2 hours. Store in an airtight container in the refrigerator for up to 2 weeks or in the freezer for up to 6 months.

CHOCOLATE PEANUT BUTTER CUP FAT BOMBS

Serves 12

Peanut butter cups are one of America's favorite candies, but packaged options are not appropriate for a keto diet. This version lets you enjoy the traditional taste without all of the carbs.

NET CARBS
5g

Calories: 209
Fat: 18g
Sodium: 4mg
Carbohydrates: 11g
Fiber: 4g
Sugar: 3g
Sugar alcohols: 2g
Protein: 6g

INGREDIENTS

½ cup Wildly Organic Coconut Butter

1 cup no-sugar-added creamy peanut butter

¼ cup raw cacao powder

2 tablespoons Swerve Brown sweetener

2 tablespoons chopped peanuts

1. Line twelve cups of a mini muffin pan with paper liners, or use a mini silicone muffin pan without liners. Set aside.

2. Combine coconut butter and peanut butter in a small saucepan over low heat. Stir until melted and smooth.

3. Stir in cacao powder and sweetener until combined. Remove from heat and fold in peanuts.

4. Pour equal amounts of mixture into twelve cups of the prepared muffin pan.

5. Transfer to refrigerator and chill until set, about 2 hours. Store in an airtight container in the refrigerator for up to 2 weeks or in the freezer for up to 6 months.

DILL PICKLE FAT BOMBS

Serves 12

Next time you empty a jar of pickles, save the juice! It adds a delicious flavor to these Dill Pickle Fat Bombs, and you can use it as a natural electrolyte-replacement drink.

Calories: 105
Fat: 10g
Sodium: 179mg
Carbohydrates: 2g
Fiber: 0g
Sugar: 1g
Sugar alcohols: 0g
Protein: 3g

INGREDIENTS

½ cup finely chopped Woodstock Organic Kosher Dill Pickles

8 ounces cream cheese, softened

1 tablespoon dill pickle juice (from a jar of Woodstock Organic Kosher Dill Pickles)

1 cup shredded Cheddar cheese

½ teaspoon garlic powder

1. Combine all ingredients in a medium bowl and beat with a handheld electric mixer on medium speed until smooth.

2. Transfer to refrigerator and chill for 30 minutes.

3. Shape mixture into twelve equal-sized balls and arrange in an airtight container. Refrigerate for 2 hours before serving.

4. Store in the refrigerator for up to 1 week.

MINT CHOCOLATE FAT BOMBS

Serves 12

If you want to bump up the amount of CLA in these fat bombs, use grass-fed butter in place of the coconut oil.

Calories: 95
Fat: 9g
Sodium: 0mg
Carbohydrates: 4g
Fiber: 3g
Sugar: 1g
Sugar alcohols: 0g
Protein: 0g

INGREDIENTS

½ cup Wildly Organic Coconut Butter

2 tablespoons coconut oil

½ teaspoon peppermint extract

¼ cup raw cacao

6 drops liquid stevia

1. Line twelve cups of a mini muffin pan with paper liners.

2. Combine all ingredients in a saucepan over low heat. Stir until melted and smooth.

3. Pour equal amounts of mixture into twelve cups of the prepared muffin pan.

4. Refrigerate until set, about 2 hours. Store in an airtight container in the refrigerator for up to 2 weeks or in the freezer for up to 6 months.

CHAPTER 11

SWEETS AND TREATS

CHOCOLATE-COVERED BACON

Serves 3

Bacon and keto-friendly chocolate? Yes, please! This Chocolate-Covered Bacon requires only four ingredients, and it satisfies both your sweet and salty cravings.

Calories: 173
Fat: 13g
Sodium: 698mg
Carbohydrates: 11g
Fiber: 6g
Sugar: 1g
Sugar alcohols: 4g
Protein: 8g

INGREDIENTS

6 slices Applegate Naturals No Sugar Bacon

¼ cup Lily's Dark Chocolate Baking Chips

2 teaspoons Perfect Keto Pure MCT Oil

½ teaspoon sea salt flakes

1. Preheat oven to 375°F. Line a baking sheet with parchment paper. Line a plate with paper towels. Set both aside.

2. Arrange bacon slices in a single layer on prepared baking sheet. Bake for 10 minutes. Flip bacon, then cook for another 10 minutes or until crispy. Remove from oven and transfer bacon to prepared plate, making sure bacon stays flat.

3. Combine baking chips and MCT oil in a small saucepan. Heat over low heat, stirring constantly, until chocolate is melted and smooth, about 5 minutes.

4. Line baking sheet with a fresh piece of parchment paper and arrange cooked bacon in a single layer on baking sheet.

5. Spoon equal amounts of melted chocolate onto each bacon strip. Sprinkle salt on top.

6. Allow chocolate to harden at room temperature about 30 minutes, then serve immediately.

CINNAMON MUG CAKE

Serves 1

When a sweet craving hits, this Cinnamon Mug Cake is ready in under 5 minutes. And since it serves only one, you won't have any leftovers and you can eat a different dessert another day.

Calories: 468
Fat: 42g
Sodium: 572mg
Carbohydrates: 20g
Fiber: 5g
Sugar: 3g
Sugar alcohols: 12g
Protein: 12g

INGREDIENTS

3 tablespoons almond flour

1 tablespoon coconut flour

1 tablespoon Swerve Granular sweetener

½ teaspoon baking powder

¼ teaspoon ground cinnamon

⅛ teaspoon sea salt

1 large egg, lightly beaten

1 tablespoon unsalted grass-fed butter, melted

3 tablespoons grass-fed heavy cream

½ teaspoon vanilla extract

1. Combine almond flour, coconut flour, sweetener, baking powder, cinnamon, and salt in a 12-ounce microwave-safe mug and mix well.

2. Add remaining ingredients and stir until combined.

3. Microwave on high for 90 seconds or until cake is set but still moist.

4. Allow to cool for 5 minutes, then serve warm.

GRANULATED OR CONFECTIONER'S?

As you've gone through these recipes, you may have noticed that some call for granulated erythritol (like the Swerve brand sweetener), while others call for confectioner's. That's because the confectioner's version dissolves more thoroughly than the granulated. You can use the two interchangeably, but if you use confectioner's instead of granulated, scale back on the amount a little bit. If you don't have confectioner's erythritol, you can make some by putting granulated erythritol in a high-speed blender and blending it until a fine powder forms.

CHOCOLATE CHIP CHAFFLES

NET CARBS
5g

Serves 2 (Makes 4 [4"] chaffles)

The mozzarella cheese in these Chocolate Chip Chaffles provides a chewy texture but such a mild flavor that you can't even taste it over the vanilla and chocolate chips.

Calories: 415
Fat: 33g
Sodium: 336mg
Carbohydrates: 44g
Fiber: 9g
Sugar: 4g
Sugar alcohols: 30g
Protein: 17g

INGREDIENTS

2 ounces cream cheese, softened

¼ cup Swerve Granular sweetener

2 large eggs

1 teaspoon vanilla extract

2 tablespoons almond flour

½ cup shredded whole milk mozzarella cheese

¼ cup Lily's Dark Chocolate Baking Chips

1. Preheat a mini waffle maker.

2. Combine cream cheese and sweetener in a medium bowl and beat with a handheld electric mixer on medium speed until smooth. Beat in eggs and vanilla until incorporated.

3. Add flour and mix until smooth. Stir in mozzarella cheese and chocolate chips.

4. Pour one-fourth of batter into heated waffle maker. Cook for 3 minutes or until steam no longer comes out of waffle maker. Repeat with remaining batter.

VANILLA MATCHA CHIA PUDDING

NET CARBS
5g

Serves 1

Keep in mind: When it comes to matcha flavor, a little goes a long way!

Calories: 221
Fat: 15g
Sodium: 63mg
Carbohydrates: 25g
Fiber: 12g
Sugar: 2g
Sugar alcohols: 8g
Protein: 7g

INGREDIENTS

3 tablespoons chia seeds

¼ cup full-fat coconut milk

¼ cup unsweetened vanilla almond milk

¼ teaspoon vanilla extract

1 teaspoon Perfect Keto Vanilla MCT Oil Powder

¼ teaspoon matcha green tea powder

2 teaspoons Swerve Brown sweetener

1. Combine all ingredients in a 16-ounce widemouthed Mason jar.

2. Shake vigorously and refrigerate for 4 hours or until pudding has set. Serve cold.

PISTACHIO FUDGE

Serves 16

This fudge holds up really well in both the refrigerator and the freezer, so don't be afraid to double the batch. You can keep it in the refrigerator for up to 2 weeks and the freezer for up to 6 months.

NET CARBS

1g

Calories: 110
Fat: 11g
Sodium: 24mg
Carbohydrates: 4g
Fiber: 1g
Sugar: 1g
Sugar alcohols: 2g
Protein: 1g

INGREDIENTS

- 9 tablespoons unsalted grass-fed butter, softened
- 4 ounces cream cheese, softened
- 3 tablespoons cacao powder
- 2 tablespoons Swerve Granular sweetener
- 1 teaspoon vanilla extract
- ½ cup shelled raw pistachio pieces, unsalted

1. Line an 8" × 8" baking pan with parchment paper and set aside.

2. Combine butter and cream cheese together in a medium bowl. Beat with a handheld electric mixer on medium speed until smooth. Add cacao powder, sweetener, and vanilla, and stir to combine. Fold in pistachio pieces.

3. Press evenly into prepared pan. Place in the refrigerator and allow to chill for 1 hour.

4. Remove from refrigerator and cut into sixteen equal-sized pieces. Store in refrigerator in airtight container until ready to serve.

STRAWBERRY CHEESECAKE BITES

Serves 6

An easy way to core a strawberry is to slice off the stem and push a stem through the top of the berry, similar to the way an apple corer works. If you prefer to eat the whole berry, you can simply slice off the stem without coring first. Once assembled, these strawberry bites will stay fresh in the refrigerator for three days.

Calories: 101
Fat: 9g
Sodium: 62mg
Carbohydrates: 11g
Fiber: 0g
Sugar: 2g
Sugar alcohols: 8g
Protein: 2g

INGREDIENTS

4 ounces cream cheese, softened

3 tablespoons grass-fed heavy cream

⅓ cup Swerve Confectioners sweetener

1 teaspoon vanilla extract

18 large whole fresh strawberries, cored and stems removed

1. Combine cream cheese and heavy cream in a medium bowl and beat with a handheld electric mixer on medium speed until smooth. Add sweetener and beat until smooth. Stir in vanilla.

2. Scoop equal amounts of cream cheese filling into each strawberry.

3. Transfer strawberries to an airtight container and refrigerate for 2 hours before serving.

STRAWBERRIES: NATURE'S SWEETS

Fruit isn't a foundation of the keto diet, but you can work in a small amount of low-sugar options, like strawberries. While strawberries do contain natural sugar in the form of fructose, a full cup contributes only 8.2 net grams of carbohydrates. Strawberries also offer loads of antioxidants, phytochemicals, vitamin C, and manganese, which can help fight off free radicals, reduce inflammation, and boost your immune system. When including fresh strawberries in your keto diet, just be mindful of your portions and don't overdo it.

FUDGY CREAM CHEESE BROWNIES

Serves 12

These Fudgy Cream Cheese Brownies are even better the next day. Whip up a batch and let them cool at room temperature overnight, then enjoy them for a snack or dessert.

INGREDIENTS

For the brownie layers:

½ cup unsalted grass-fed butter

⅔ cup Swerve Confectioners sweetener

½ cup raw cacao powder

½ teaspoon sea salt

2 large eggs

2 tablespoons grass-fed heavy cream

¾ cup almond flour

For the cheesecake layer:

8 ounces cream cheese, softened

¼ cup Swerve Confectioners sweetener

1 large egg

1 teaspoon vanilla extract

1. Preheat oven to 350°F. Line an 8" × 8" baking pan with parchment paper and set aside.

2. To make the brownie layers, heat butter in a medium saucepan over medium-low heat. When melted, add sweetener and stir until dissolved, about 2 minutes. Stir in cacao powder and salt. Remove from heat and allow to cool slightly.

3. Add eggs one at a time, whisking quickly to incorporate them into the mixture. Whisk in cream and then stir in flour.

4. Transfer two-thirds of the mixture to prepared baking pan and spread evenly. Set the rest aside.

5. To make the cheesecake layer, combine cream cheese and sweetener in a medium bowl and beat with a handheld electric mixer on medium speed until smooth. Beat in egg and vanilla.

6. Spread cream cheese mixture on top of brownie layer. Scoop the remaining brownie batter on top of cream cheese layer and use a knife to create a swirl pattern.

7. Bake for 20 minutes or until brownies are set. Remove from oven and allow to cool completely before serving.

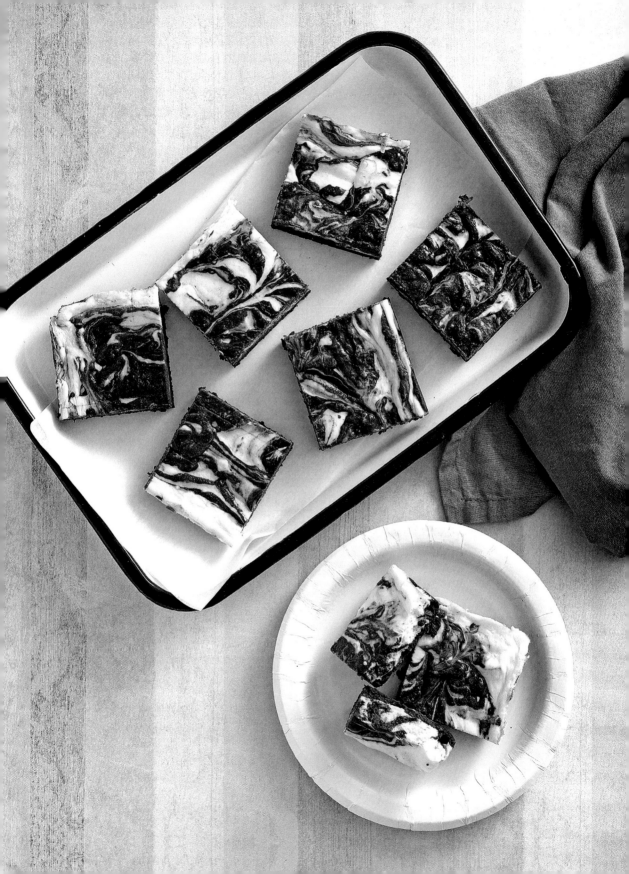

COOKIES AND CREAM DESSERT WAFFLES

NET CARBS
7g

Calories: 430
Fat: 38g
Sodium: 459mg
Carbohydrates: 55g
Fiber: 6g
Sugar: 4g
Sugar alcohols: 42g
Protein: 10g

Serves 2 (Makes 2 [4"] sandwiched waffles)

These Cookies and Cream Dessert Waffles taste just like those popular sandwich cookies but without any of the refined sugar or artificial ingredients. If you have a few net carbs to spare, you can drizzle some ChocZero Chocolate Syrup on top before serving.

INGREDIENTS

For the waffles:

3 tablespoons raw cacao powder

3½ tablespoons Swerve Granular sweetener

1½ tablespoons grass-fed heavy cream

1 large egg, lightly beaten

¾ teaspoon vanilla extract

½ teaspoon baking powder

⅛ teaspoon sea salt

2 tablespoons Lily's Dark Chocolate Baking Chips

For the filling:

4 ounces cream cheese, softened

¼ cup Swerve Confectioners sweetener

2 tablespoons grass-fed heavy cream

¼ teaspoon vanilla extract

1. Preheat a mini waffle maker.

2. To make the waffles, combine cacao powder, granular sweetener, cream, egg, vanilla, baking powder, salt, and chocolate chips in a small bowl, and stir to combine.

3. Pour one-fourth of batter into heated waffle maker. Cook for 3 minutes or until steam no longer comes out of waffle maker. Remove from waffle maker and repeat with remaining batter.

4. To make the filling, combine filling ingredients in a medium bowl and beat with a handheld electric mixture on low speed until smooth.

5. Scoop half of filling onto each of two waffles. Top with remaining waffles, and serve.

MINT CHOCOLATE BITES

Serves 5 (Makes 10 bites)

These Mint Chocolate Bites are the perfect after-dinner treat, but they're also a perfectly balanced fat bomb. You can save them for dessert or eat them as a snack on days when you feel a little more hungry than usual.

NET CARBS
2g

Calories: 216
Fat: 20g
Sodium: 1mg
Carbohydrates: 34g
Fiber: 6g
Sugar: 2g
Sugar alcohols: 26g
Protein: 2g

INGREDIENTS

¼ cup coconut oil

¾ cup Swerve Confectioners sweetener

1 teaspoon peppermint extract

2 teaspoons grass-fed heavy cream

½ cup Lily's Dark Chocolate Baking Chips

2 teaspoons Nutiva Organic Coconut Oil with Buttery Flavor

1. Place a wire baking rack on a baking sheet. Set aside.

2. Combine coconut oil, sweetener, peppermint, and cream in a medium bowl and beat with a handheld electric mixer on medium speed until smooth. Refrigerate for 10 minutes.

3. Form mixture into ten balls and place on wire rack.

4. Combine chocolate chips and coconut oil in a small saucepan over low heat. Heat until chocolate melts and oil is evenly incorporated, stirring frequently, about 5 minutes.

5. Remove from heat and carefully pour chocolate evenly over each ball to coat. Transfer baking sheet to the refrigerator and refrigerate for 2 hours until set.

PUMPKIN CINNAMON ROLL COFFEE CAKE

Serves 12

Pumpkin gets a lot of attention in October, but it's divine any time of the year, especially in this keto coffee cake. Make sure you're purchasing pumpkin purée, which contains only pumpkin, not pumpkin pie filling, which has added sugar and a higher carb count.

INGREDIENTS

For the cake:

2 cups almond flour

1 cup Swerve Granular sweetener

3 teaspoons pumpkin pie spice

2 teaspoons baking powder

¼ teaspoon baking soda

½ teaspoon sea salt

½ cup unsalted grass-fed butter, melted

¼ cup sour cream

2 large eggs

¾ cup pumpkin purée

1 teaspoon vanilla extract

For the crumb topping:

1 cup almond flour

½ cup Swerve Granular sweetener

½ cup coconut flour

½ cup crushed walnuts

2 teaspoons pumpkin pie spice

⅛ teaspoon sea salt

½ cup unsalted grass-fed butter, chilled and cubed

1. Preheat oven to 350°F. Grease a 9" × 9" baking dish with grass-fed butter and set aside.

2. To make the cake, combine almond flour, sweetener, pumpkin pie spice, baking powder, baking soda, and salt in a large bowl. Mix well.

3. Combine melted butter, sour cream, eggs, pumpkin purée, and vanilla in a separate medium bowl and mix well. Fold pumpkin mixture into flour mixture and mix until just incorporated. Transfer to prepared baking dish.

4. To make the crumb topping, combine almond flour, sweetener, coconut flour, walnuts, pumpkin pie spice, and salt in a medium bowl. Cut chilled butter into the mixture with a fork or pastry cutter until crumbly.

5. Sprinkle crumb mixture evenly over the top of the cake batter. Bake 30 minutes or until a toothpick inserted in the center comes out clean.

6. Remove from oven and allow to cool for 1 hour, then cut into twelve equal-sized portions and serve.

CHOCOLATE CHIP CHEESECAKE DIP

Serves 12

Keto-friendly graham crackers are hard to find, but you can use Catalina Crunch Honey Graham or Cinnamon Toast cereal pieces to scoop up this dip. If you don't have any, simply eat it with a spoon!

NET CARBS
3g

Calories: 227
Fat: 21g
Sodium: 62mg
Carbohydrates: 26g
Fiber: 9g
Sugar: 2g
Sugar alcohols: 14g
Protein: 3g

INGREDIENTS

8 ounces cream cheese, softened

½ cup unsalted grass-fed butter, softened

¾ cup Swerve Confectioners sweetener

2 tablespoons Swerve Brown sweetener

½ teaspoon vanilla extract

¾ cup Lily's Milk Chocolate Style Baking Chips

½ cup crushed raw walnuts

¼ cup ChocZero Chocolate Syrup

1. Lightly grease a 9" × 5" loaf pan. Set aside.

2. Combine cream cheese and butter in a medium bowl and beat with a handheld electric mixer on medium speed until smooth. Beat in both sweeteners until incorporated. Stir in vanilla and chocolate chips.

3. Transfer mixture to prepared loaf pan. Sprinkle crushed walnuts evenly on top. Drizzle chocolate syrup over walnuts.

4. Refrigerate for 15 minutes before serving.

CHOOSING A CHOCOLATE CHIP

There are several different "sugar-free" chocolate chip options out there, but most of them contain maltitol, the sugar alcohol that has questionable effects on your blood sugar and insulin levels (and frequently causes gas, bloating, and diarrhea). It's worth the extra effort to find Lily's brand, which is sweetened with stevia and erythritol, the best sugar alcohol choice. They're now available in many grocery stores and even Walmart stores. If you can't find them in the regular aisles, check your store's health food section.

CHOCOLATE CARAMEL MUG CAKE

Serves 1

This Chocolate Caramel Mug Cake is the perfect-sized dessert for one, but if you're making it for two, just double the recipe. Mix everything in one bowl, then divide the batter equally between two separate microwave-safe mugs.

Calories: 336
Fat: 26g
Sodium: 648mg
Carbohydrates: 27g
Fiber: 18g
Sugar: 1g
Sugar alcohols: 4g
Protein: 11g

INGREDIENTS

- 3 tablespoons almond flour
- 1 tablespoon raw cacao powder
- 1 teaspoon Swerve Confectioners sweetener
- ½ teaspoon baking powder
- ¹⁄₁₆ teaspoon sea salt
- 1 large egg, lightly beaten
- 1 tablespoon unsalted grass-fed butter, melted
- 1 tablespoon ChocZero Caramel Syrup

1. Combine flour, cacao powder, sweetener, baking powder, and salt in a 12-ounce microwave-safe mug. Mix well.

2. Add egg and butter and stir until incorporated.

3. Microwave on high for 1 minute or until cake is set but still moist.

4. Remove from microwave and drizzle caramel syrup on top.

5. Allow to cool for 5 minutes, then serve warm.

CHOCOLATE CHIP NUT BUTTER FUDGE

Serves 16

Perfect Keto Nut Butter combines cashews, macadamia nuts, and coconut to form a blend of high-quality nut butter that's loaded with healthy fats and MCTs that can help boost your energy and keep you full. If you don't have any, you can substitute equal amounts of the nut butter of your choice.

NET CARBS

0g

Calories: 270
Fat: 28g
Sodium: 1mg
Carbohydrates: 8g
Fiber: 5g
Sugar: 1g
Sugar alcohols: 3g
Protein: 2g

INGREDIENTS

1 cup Perfect Keto Macadamia Vanilla Nut Butter

1 cup Nutiva Organic Coconut Oil with Buttery Flavor

¼ cup grass-fed heavy cream

1 teaspoon vanilla extract

2 tablespoons Swerve Confectioners sweetener

½ cup Lily's Dark Chocolate Baking Chips

1. Line an 8" × 8" baking dish with parchment paper and set aside.

2. Combine nut butter and coconut oil in a saucepan over medium-low heat. Heat until melted and smooth, about 3 minutes. Add cream, vanilla, and sweetener, and stir until smooth.

3. Remove from heat and allow to cool for 5 minutes before stirring in chocolate chips.

4. Pour mixture into prepared baking dish and refrigerate for 2 hours or until set.

5. Remove from pan and cut into sixteen equal squares. Store in an airtight container in refrigerator until ready to serve.

LEMON POUND CAKE

Serves 12

Don't skip the lemon zest in this pound cake! It may seem like a small addition, but it's responsible for a lot of the rich lemon flavor.

INGREDIENTS

1¼ cups almond flour

1 teaspoon baking powder

¼ teaspoon sea salt

4 tablespoons unsalted grass-fed butter, softened

¾ cup Swerve Granular sweetener

4 ounces cream cheese, softened

1 teaspoon lemon extract

2 teaspoons lemon zest

4 large eggs

1. Preheat oven to 350°F. Grease a 9" × 5" loaf pan with grass-fed butter and set aside.

2. Combine flour, baking powder, and salt in a medium bowl and set aside.

3. In a separate medium bowl, combine butter and sweetener. Beat with a handheld electric mixer on medium speed until combined and fluffy. Beat in cream cheese, lemon extract, and lemon zest until smooth. Beat eggs in one at a time.

4. Stir in flour mixture until well incorporated. Transfer to prepared loaf pan and bake for 30 minutes or until a toothpick inserted in the center comes out clean. Remove from oven and allow to cool completely before serving.

ZESTING A LEMON

When zesting a lemon, it's helpful to use a small, fine grater called a microplane. You want to zest only the yellow part of the skin and avoid the white layer underneath, which is called the pith. The pith has a bitter flavor and can be off-putting in recipes. To zest, rub the lemon against the microplane in one direction and turn the lemon as you go, so you don't get too deep.

SALTED CARAMEL CHEESECAKE

Serves 12

Thanks to companies like ChocZero, having to make your own keto-approved caramel sauce has become a thing of the past. With only 1 gram of net carbs per serving, you can even drizzle on a little extra.

Calories: 237
Fat: 22g
Sodium: 146mg
Carbohydrates: 19g
Fiber: 6g
Sugar: 2g
Sugar alcohols: 10g
Protein: 5g

INGREDIENTS

For the crust:

1 cup shelled whole raw almonds

1 tablespoon Swerve Granular sweetener

1 teaspoon ground cinnamon

¼ teaspoon ground nutmeg

2 tablespoons salted grass-fed butter, melted

For the filling:

12 ounces cream cheese, softened

¼ cup sour cream

¼ cup grass-fed heavy cream

1 tablespoon salted grass-fed butter, melted

½ cup Swerve Granular sweetener

1 large egg

1 teaspoon vanilla extract

For the topping:

¼ cup ChocZero Caramel Syrup

¼ teaspoon sea salt flakes

1. Preheat oven to 350°F. Line a 9" springform baking pan with parchment paper and set aside.

2. To make the crust, add almonds to a food processor and pulse until coarse crumbs form. Add sweetener, cinnamon, and nutmeg, and pulse to combine. Pour in butter and pulse until incorporated.

3. Transfer mixture to prepared baking pan and press down evenly into pan to form a crust. Set aside.

4. To make the filling, combine cream cheese and sour cream in a medium bowl and beat with a handheld electric mixer on medium speed until smooth. Beat in heavy cream until smooth. Add remaining ingredients and beat until smooth.

5. Pour mixture on top of crust and spread out evenly. Bake for 35 minutes or until cheesecake is set but still wobbly in the center.

6. Remove from oven and allow to cool for 5 minutes. Run a knife around the edge of the cheesecake and remove sides of springform pan. Allow to cool completely, about 2 hours.

7. Drizzle caramel sauce evenly on top of cooled cheesecake and sprinkle with salt. Refrigerate until ready to serve.

DOUBLE CHOCOLATE MOUSSE BARS

Serves 8

These Double Chocolate Mousse Bars combine a chocolate crust with rich, chocolatey mousse, but if you're short on time and looking for a quick dessert, skip the crust and just eat the mousse with a spoon.

NET CARBS
4g

Calories: 271
Fat: 26g
Sodium: 131mg
Carbohydrates: 11g
Fiber: 2g
Sugar: 2g
Sugar alcohols: 5g
Protein: 5g

INGREDIENTS

For the crust:

1 cup almond flour

2 teaspoons raw cacao powder

2 teaspoons Swerve Granular sweetener

3 tablespoons unsalted grass-fed butter, melted

For the filling:

8 ounces cream cheese, softened

½ cup grass-fed heavy cream

1 teaspoon vanilla extract

3 tablespoons raw cacao powder

¼ cup Swerve Confectioners sweetener

⅛ teaspoon sea salt

1. Line an 8" × 8" baking pan with parchment paper and set aside.

2. To make the crust, combine flour, cacao powder, and granular sweetener in a small bowl and mix well. Add melted butter and stir until incorporated.

3. Press mixture evenly into prepared baking pan, forming a crust.

4. To make the filling, combine cream cheese and heavy cream in a separate medium bowl. Beat with a handheld electric mixer on medium speed until smooth. Stir in vanilla.

5. Add remaining ingredients and beat on medium speed until light and fluffy.

6. Fold cream cheese filling onto crust and spread out evenly.

7. Refrigerate for 1 hour before cutting into bars and serving.

NO-BAKE ALMOND BUTTER COOKIES

Serves 6 (Makes 12 cookies)

NET CARBS
4g

Calories: 297
Fat: 28g
Sodium: 69mg
Carbohydrates: 15g
Fiber: 5g
Sugar: 3g
Sugar alcohols: 6g
Protein: 7g

These No-Bake Almond Butter Cookies are the perfect way to satisfy your sweet tooth in the summer months when you don't want to turn on your oven. But, because they're not baked, they melt if they get too hot. Store them in the refrigerator and take them out only when you're ready to eat them.

INGREDIENTS

2 tablespoons salted grass-fed butter

¼ cup Swerve Confectioners sweetener

⅔ cup crunchy no-sugar-added almond butter

1 tablespoon raw cacao powder

1 cup unsweetened shredded coconut

1. Line a baking sheet with parchment paper and set aside.

2. Heat butter in a small saucepan over medium-low heat. Add sweetener and stir until dissolved, about 2 minutes.

3. Add almond butter and heat until melted, about 3 minutes, stirring occasionally. When mixture is smooth, stir in cacao powder.

4. Remove from heat and add shredded coconut. Mix well.

5. Form mixture into twelve equal-sized balls and arrange on prepared baking sheet.

6. Press each ball down to form a flat cookie. Refrigerate for 1 hour or until set.

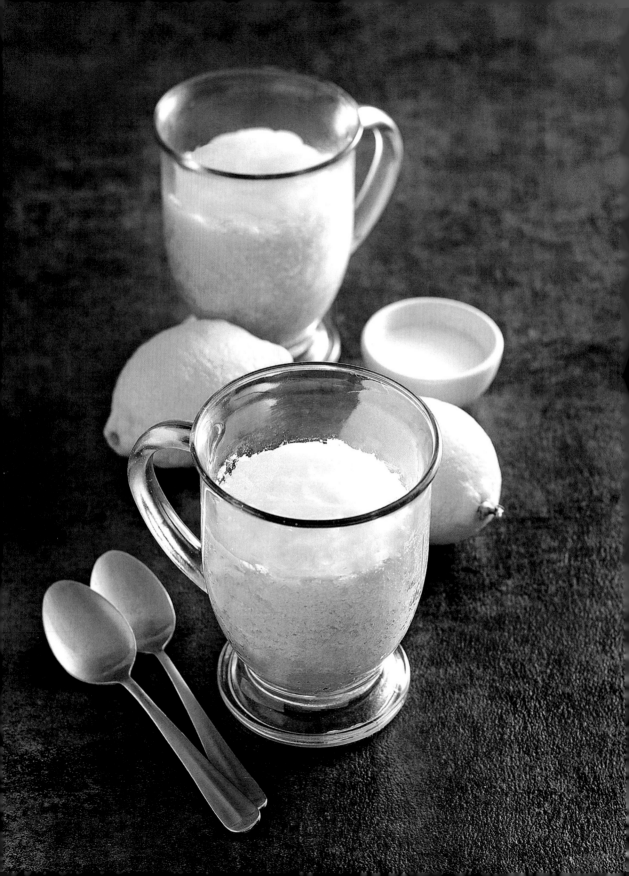

LEMON MUG CAKES WITH LEMON ICING

Serves 2

Try to use fresh lemon juice instead of the bottled stuff for this recipe—the flavor will be brighter.

INGREDIENTS

For the cake:

¾ cup almond flour

3 tablespoons Swerve Granular sweetener

½ teaspoon baking powder

⅛ teaspoon sea salt

2 tablespoons fresh lemon juice

2 teaspoons lemon zest

1 large egg, lightly beaten

2 tablespoons unsalted grass-fed butter, melted

For the icing:

2 tablespoons Swerve Confectioners sweetener

½ teaspoon water

½ teaspoon fresh lemon juice

1. To make the cake, mix flour, granular sweetener, baking powder, and salt together in a medium bowl. Add lemon juice, lemon zest, egg, and melted butter, and whisk until combined.

2. Divide mixture evenly between two 12-ounce microwave-safe mugs. Microwave on high for 90 seconds each or until cakes are set but still moist.

3. To make the icing, mix sweetener, water, and lemon juice together in a small bowl until smooth. Drizzle icing mixture on top of each mug cake.

4. Serve warm.

CHOCOLATE CHIP COOKIE DOUGH BITES

Serves 12 (Makes 24 bites)

Lots of people can agree that the cookie dough is the best part of the cookie. With these Chocolate Chip Cookie Dough Bites, you'll get all the warm fuzzies that come with raw cookie dough but without any of the refined sugar or raw eggs.

NET CARBS

2g

Calories: 201
Fat: 19g
Sodium: 157mg
Carbohydrates: 17g
Fiber: 4g
Sugar: 2g
Sugar alcohols: 11g
Protein: 3g

INGREDIENTS

8 ounces cream cheese, softened

½ cup unsalted grass-fed butter, softened

2 teaspoons vanilla extract

¼ cup almond flour

½ cup Swerve Granular sweetener

½ teaspoon sea salt

⅔ cup Lily's Dark Chocolate Baking Chips

1. Line a baking sheet with parchment paper and set aside.

2. Combine cream cheese and butter in a medium bowl and beat with a handheld electric mixer on medium speed until light and fluffy.

3. Stir in vanilla.

4. In a separate small bowl, combine flour, sweetener, and salt. Gradually mix into cream cheese mixture. Stir in chocolate chips.

5. Refrigerate for 30 minutes or until hardened.

6. Form mixture into twenty-four one-inch balls and arrange on prepared baking sheet. Refrigerate for 2 hours.

7. Store in an airtight container in the refrigerator until ready to serve.

DARK CHOCOLATE CHOCOLATE CHIP ICE CREAM

NET CARBS
9g

Calories: 747
Fat: 68g
Sodium: 141mg
Carbohydrates: 80g
Fiber: 20g
Sugar: 9g
Sugar alcohols: 51g
Protein: 12g

Serves 4

Who says you have to get rid of chocolate on a keto diet? This Dark Chocolate Chocolate Chip Ice Cream satisfies your chocolate craving with just a few bites and only a few net carbs per serving. You'll need an ice cream maker for this recipe.

INGREDIENTS

2 large eggs

1 cup Swerve Confectioners sweetener

2 cups grass-fed heavy cream

1 teaspoon vanilla extract

⅛ teaspoon sea salt

¾ cup plus ½ cup Lily's Dark Chocolate Baking Chips, divided

1. Place eggs in a medium bowl and beat with a handheld electric mixer on high speed until foamy. Gradually add sweetener and beat until incorporated. Set aside.

2. Combine cream, vanilla, and salt in a medium saucepan over low heat. Slowly add eggs, whisking constantly. Continue whisking for 2 minutes.

3. Remove from heat and stir in ¾ cup chocolate chips. Continue stirring until chocolate melts and mixture is smooth, about 5 minutes. Refrigerate mixture for 30 minutes.

4. Pour chilled mixture into ice cream maker and allow to cool for 5 minutes.

5. Stir in remaining chocolate chips and follow manufacturer's instructions for preparing ice cream.

6. Serve frozen.

MEAL PLANS

WEEK 1

Monday	Net Carbs
Breakfast: Eggs Florentine	1g
Lunch: Spaghetti Squash Spinach Alfredo	8g
Snack: Buffalo Chicken Celery Boats	2g
Dinner: Stuffed Pork Tenderloin with Fried Shaved Brussels Sprouts	2g + 3g
Dessert: Cinnamon Mug Cake	3g
Total Net Carbs:	**19g**
Tuesday	Net Carbs
Breakfast: Sausage Cream Cheese Pinwheels	3g
Lunch: Ground Turkey and Zucchini Rice Bowl	6g
Snack: Bacon and Chive–Stuffed Tomatoes	3g
Dinner: Lamb Chops with Mint Butter and Garlic-Roasted Mushrooms	1g + 2g
Dessert: Salted Caramel Cheesecake	3g
Total Net Carbs:	**18g**
Wednesday	Net Carbs
Breakfast: Cheesy Spinach Quiche	3g
Lunch: Spicy Sausage Burrito Bowls	4g
Snack: Spicy Pimento Cheese Dip	2g
Dinner: Salmon Piccata with Roasted Garlic and Lemon Broccoli	5g + 3g
Dessert: Chocolate-Covered Bacon	1g
Total Net Carbs:	**18g**
Thursday	Net Carbs
Breakfast: Jalapeño Cheddar Chaffles	1g
Lunch: Kale and Avocado Salad	4g
Snack: Savory Herb Chaffles	5g
Dinner: Egg Roll Skillet	5g
Dessert: Strawberry Cheesecake Bites	3g
Total Net Carbs:	**18g**

Friday	Net Carbs
Breakfast: Everything Bagels	6g
Lunch: Creamy Broccoli and Cauliflower Soup	4g
Snack: Fried Pickles	2g
Dinner: Parmesan and Herb–Crusted Turkey Tenderloin with Garlic Butter–Roasted Cauliflower	0g + 4g
Dessert: Chocolate Chip Cheesecake Dip	3g
Total Net Carbs:	**19g**
Saturday	Net Carbs
Breakfast: Chocolate Chip Muffins	3g
Lunch: Creamy Chicken and Bacon Soup	4g
Snack: Pizza Bites	1g
Dinner: Roasted Leg of Lamb with Maple-Roasted Brussels Sprouts	1g + 4g
Dessert: Chocolate Caramel Mug Cake	5g
Total Net Carbs:	**18g**
Sunday	Net Carbs
Breakfast: Cinnamon Waffles with Cinnamon Cream Cheese Icing	4g
Lunch: Salmon-Stuffed Avocado	3g
Snack: Cheesy Taco Dip	3g
Dinner: Butter Steak with Garlic and Chives and Pan-Glazed Mushrooms	1g + 4g
Dessert: Double Chocolate Mousse Bars	4g
Total Net Carbs:	**19g**

WEEK 2

Monday	Net Carbs
Breakfast: Maple and Brown Sugar Porridge	6g
Lunch: Greek Zoodle Salad	6g
Snack: Spiced Roasted Pumpkin Seeds	1g
Dinner: Baked Lemon Garlic Salmon with Herb-Roasted Asparagus	2g + 1g
Dessert: Fudgy Cream Cheese Brownies	2g
Total Net Carbs:	**18g**
Tuesday	Net Carbs
Breakfast: Bacon Cheddar Chive Biscuits	3g
Lunch: Crab Endive Cups	1g
Snack: Chicken Parmesan Dip	2g
Dinner: Turkey Bacon Cheeseburger Meatloaf with Jalapeño Popper Mashed Cauliflower	4g + 7g
Dessert: Chocolate Chip Nut Butter Fudge	0g
Total Net Carbs:	**17g**

Wednesday	Net Carbs
Breakfast: Buffalo Chicken Egg Cups	0g
Lunch: Jalapeño Cheddar Soup	5g
Snack: Baked Chicken Wings	3g
Dinner: Beef Carnitas with Fresh Broccoli Slaw	1g + 2g
Dessert: Cookies and Cream Dessert Waffles	7g
Total Net Carbs:	**18g**
Thursday	**Net Carbs**
Breakfast: Blueberry Almond Overnight "Oats"	5g
Lunch: Decadent Crab Cakes	4g
Snack: Cheesy Ranch Cauliflower Bites	4g
Dinner: White Chicken Chili	4g
Dessert: Mint Chocolate Bites	2g
Total Net Carbs:	**19g**
Friday	**Net Carbs**
Breakfast: Kale and Eggs	3g
Lunch: Bacon Turkey Club Mason Jar Salad	4g
Snack: Maple-Roasted Almonds	3g
Dinner: Parmesan-Crusted Pork Chops with Breadless Broccoli Gratin	2g + 5g
Dessert: Chocolate Chip Cookie Dough Bites	2g
Total Net Carbs:	**19g**
Saturday	**Net Carbs**
Breakfast: Bacon and Egg Cheese Sandwich	3g
Lunch: Beef Curry	3g
Snack: Sausage and Cheese Bites	0g
Dinner: Grilled Lamb Burgers with Parmesan Rainbow Chard	2g + 6g
Dessert: Lemon Mug Cakes with Lemon Icing	5g
Total Net Carbs:	**19g**
Sunday	**Net Carbs**
Breakfast: Maple Bacon Mini Waffles	3g
Lunch: Deconstructed Stuffed Pepper Bowls	7g
Snack: Chile con Queso	1g
Dinner: Garlic-Crusted Chicken Thighs with Roasted Okra	3g + 3g
Dessert: Pistachio Fudge	1g
Total Net Carbs:	**18g**

PANTRY STAPLES

OILS, BUTTERS, FATS, AND SAUCES

Avocado oil

Avocado oil cooking spray

Canned (full-fat) coconut milk

ChocZero Caramel Syrup

ChocZero Maple Syrup

Cholula Original Hot Sauce

Coconut aminos

Coconut oil

Coconut oil cooking spray

Frank's RedHot Original Cayenne Pepper Sauce

Kettle & Fire Classic Beef Bone Broth

Kettle & Fire Classic Chicken Bone Broth

Macadamia nut butter

Nature's Promise Organic Sesame Tahini

The New Primal Hot Buffalo Sauce

No-sugar-added sunflower seed butter

Nutiva Organic Coconut Oil with Buttery Flavor

Nutiva Organic Liquid Coconut Oil with Garlic

Perfect Keto Nut Butter (various flavors)

Primal Kitchen Classic BBQ Sauce, Organic and Unsweetened

Primal Kitchen Italian Vinaigrette & Marinade

Rao's Homemade Marinara Sauce

Tessemae's Organic Mayonnaise

Tessemae's Organic Ranch dressings

Tessemae's Unsweetened Ketchup

Wildbrine Spicy Kimchi Sriracha sauce

Wildly Organic Coconut Butter

SUGAR SUBSTITUTES AND CHOCOLATE

Good Dee's Sugar-Free Sprinkles

Lily's chocolate baking chips

Liquid stevia

SweetLeaf Sweet Drops Caramel Flavored Stevia Sweetener

SweetLeaf Sweet Drops Chocolate Flavored Stevia Sweetener

Swerve Brown sweetener

Swerve Confectioners sweetener

Swerve Granular sweetener

EXTRACTS

Almond extract

Lemon extract

Peppermint extract

Vanilla extract

FLOURS, SEEDS, SEASONINGS, AND POWDERS

Almond flour

Almond meal

Arrowroot powder

California Gold Dust Superspice Mix

Chia seeds

Coconut flour

EPIC Oven Baked Pink Himalayan and Sea Salt Pork Rinds

Good Dee's Cracker Biscuit Mix

Ground flaxseed meal (or whole flax)

Hemp hearts

Herbes de Provence seasoning

Matcha green tea powder

McCormick Grill Mates Montreal Steak Seasoning

McCormick Old Bay Seasoning

Perfect Keto MCT Oil Powder (chocolate and vanilla)

Raw cacao powder

Sea salt flakes

Trader Joe's Everything But the Bagel Sesame Seasoning Blend

Xanthan gum

MEAT AND SEAFOOD

Canned white chunk chicken breast

Canned wild Alaskan pink salmon

Canned wild-caught lump crabmeat

HELPFUL APPLIANCES AND KITCHEN TOOLS

Air fryer

Dash mini waffle maker

Food processor

Handheld electric mixer

High-speed blender

Ice cream maker

Instant Pot® pressure cooker

Mandoline slicer

Mini muffin tins and/or silicone baking molds

Parchment paper and/or silicone baking mats

Slow cooker

Vegetable spiralizer

STANDARD US/METRIC MEASUREMENT CONVERSIONS

VOLUME CONVERSIONS

US Volume Measure	Metric Equivalent
⅛ teaspoon	0.5 milliliter
¼ teaspoon	1 milliliter
½ teaspoon	2 milliliters
1 teaspoon	5 milliliters
½ tablespoon	7 milliliters
1 tablespoon (3 teaspoons)	15 milliliters
2 tablespoons (1 fluid ounce)	30 milliliters
¼ cup (4 tablespoons)	60 milliliters
⅓ cup	90 milliliters
½ cup (4 fluid ounces)	125 milliliters
⅔ cup	160 milliliters
¾ cup (6 fluid ounces)	180 milliliters
1 cup (16 tablespoons)	250 milliliters
1 pint (2 cups)	500 milliliters
1 quart (4 cups)	1 liter (about)

WEIGHT CONVERSIONS

US Weight Measure	Metric Equivalent
½ ounce	15 grams
1 ounce	30 grams
2 ounces	60 grams
3 ounces	85 grams
¼ pound (4 ounces)	115 grams
½ pound (8 ounces)	225 grams
¾ pound (12 ounces)	340 grams
1 pound (16 ounces)	454 grams

OVEN TEMPERATURE CONVERSIONS

Degrees Fahrenheit	Degrees Celsius
200 degrees F	95 degrees C
250 degrees F	120 degrees C
275 degrees F	135 degrees C
300 degrees F	150 degrees C
325 degrees F	160 degrees C
350 degrees F	180 degrees C
375 degrees F	190 degrees C
400 degrees F	205 degrees C
425 degrees F	220 degrees C
450 degrees F	230 degrees C

BAKING PAN SIZES

American	Metric
8 x 1½ inch round baking pan	20 x 4 cm cake tin
9 x 1½ inch round baking pan	23 x 3.5 cm cake tin
11 x 7 x 1½ inch baking pan	28 x 18 x 4 cm baking tin
13 x 9 x 2 inch baking pan	30 x 20 x 5 cm baking tin
2 quart rectangular baking dish	30 x 20 x 3 cm baking tin
15 x 10 x 2 inch baking pan	30 x 25 x 2 cm baking tin (Swiss roll tin)
9 inch pie plate	22 x 4 or 23 x 4 cm pie plate
7 or 8 inch springform pan	18 or 20 cm springform or loose bottom cake tin
9 x 5 x 3 inch loaf pan	23 x 13 x 7 cm or 2 lb narrow loaf or pâté tin
1½ quart casserole	1.5 liter casserole
2 quart casserole	2 liter casserole

INDEX

Note: Page numbers in **bold** indicate recipe category lists.

ABOUT THE AUTHOR

LINDSAY BOYERS, CHNC, is a holistic nutritionist with extensive experience in a wide range of dietary therapies, including the ketogenic diet. She specializes in gut health, mood disorders, and functional nutrition. Lindsay has a degree in food and nutrition from Framingham State University and is certified in both holistic and functional nutrition. She lives in Shrewsbury, Massachusetts.